CW00927312

The Gout Handbook

Everything you need to know

Ben Jones &
David G Hansen

The Pocket Doctor

Published by

The Pocket Doctor

An imprint of Birch Briar Media

thepocketdoctor.org

Published 2022

Disclaimer

This Handbook contains general information relating to various medical conditions and their treatment. Such information is provided for informational purposes only and is not meant to be a substitute for advice provided by a doctor or other qualified health care professional. You should not use the information contained herein for diagnosing a health problem or disease. You should always consult with a doctor or other health care professional for medical advice or information about diagnosis and treatment.

British Library Cataloguing in Publication Data: Available on request.

Library of Congress Control Number: Available on request

ISBN 978-1-73-958132-9

Preface to The Pocket Doctor series

The seeds that would lead to this new series of medical handbooks for patients were sown in different places and times. A powerful moment of inspiration came in a car dealership as the mechanic explained in baffling technical terms what was wrong with Ben's car and why it would be so expensive to fix. He realised that many of his patients must feel the same way. He began to think more carefully about how to explain complex medical issues in ways clear and understandable to the layperson.

Some years later, to pay the bills whilst toiling over his PhD thesis, Ben took a part-time job as a medical escort, flying around the world to bring home people who had become ill while overseas and who could not fly without a doctor to accompany them. Typically, they would spend twelve to twenty-four hours together. With this came the luxury of lots of time for the patient and travelling family members to ask Ben all the questions they could think of regarding the patient's ailments and the future implications. It was an opportunity everyone greatly appreciated.

Later still, David and Ben compared their experiences of coaching friends, family members and acquaintances to ensure they got the correct diagnosis and treatment from other doctors, explaining which symptoms to draw attention to and what questions to ask. Later they'd spend time answering the questions those individuals had not thought to ask their doctors or hadn't had the time to ask.

From all these experiences, the idea of this series was born. To create a series of handbooks that provide comprehensive information to allow patients to truly understand the disease that affects them, talk knowledgeably with their doctors, take an active part in their own care, and share in decision-making.

All too often, we can feel anxious, scared and helpless when confronted with the diagnosis of a serious and/or complex disease. Our sincere hope is that these handbooks will give you the knowledge and confidence you need to overcome that feeling of helplessness, and to work with your doctors and other healthcare providers for the best possible outcomes.

One last but crucial point: The human body is hugely complex, diseases don't always behave as the medical textbooks say they should, and conditions and drugs interact. Doctors spend years learning their craft and their whole lifetimes refining it. There is no substitute for the expert opinion of your doctor. The purpose of these handbooks is to enable you to make the most effective use of the time with your doctor, not to replace it.

Preface to The Gout Handbook

Having gout is no joke. Joint pain during a flare-up can be excruciating, making it impossible to work or do normal activities. One in five individuals with gout will also develop kidney stones, another opportunity for incapacitating pain. In the long term, permanent joint damage can result.

Diagnosis is not always straightforward. Other conditions give similar symptoms, yet an accurate diagnosis is essential for appropriate treatment. Many treatment choices are available, each with pros and cons. Optimizing treatment often requires regular monitoring. Given all this complexity, it's not surprising that most people with gout are not on optimal treatment.

Getting the best treatment requires a close working relationship between patient and doctor, but this is not the norm. Typically, the patient lacks sufficient knowledge to participate actively in decisions about their treatment. This lack of knowledge, coupled with consultations that often feel rushed, means there's little discussion, so doctors make decisions without understanding their patient's perspective. All this can leave the patient feeling helpless and with little control over their treatment.

The Gout Handbook aims to change that. Providing information clearly and straightforwardly and aimed squarely at the patient's perspective and needs, The Gout Handbook helps you to really understand your gout. The Handbook leads you through all aspects of the condition and acts as a reference you can turn to with all your questions. Case histories help you learn through real-world examples. They let you try your hand at clinical decision making and, together with quizzes, reinforce your understanding.

The Handbook ends with a personal data section. Here you can record the details of the condition as it affects you. There are specially designed tables, charts and forms, and space to note the questions you'd like to discuss with your doctor at your next visit.

Armed with knowledge and facts, you will be confident to discuss the issues with your doctor, and be fully involved in decisions about your care. You won't need to feel helpless and wholly dependent on your doctor.

Our website and newsletter provide breaking news of medical advances; clinical trials; interviews with doctors, patients, and researchers; updates to the Handbook, and much more. Please visit us there and share your thoughts on The Gout Handbook. Tell us what you like and what you'd like us to do differently. If you have questions we haven't answered, please let us know so we can include them in the next edition. We want you to get the best medical care possible, and we want The Gout Handbook to be the best resource to help you achieve that goal.

Contents

Chapter 1

Gout in a nutshell

You can use this chapter as a quick overview of gout for yourself or for family members who want to know the basics without reading the whole book.

Gout is a type of arthritis that occurs when crystals of a chemical called monosodium urate form in joints. It can affect various joints, including the feet, ankles, knees, wrists, and elbows, but the big toes are those most commonly affected. Typically, the pain is very severe, comes on rapidly, and the affected joint is tender, red, and swollen. There may also be fever, chills, and a general feeling of being unwell.

Attacks may occur several times a year and usually settle on their own in a few days. As time goes by, the attacks may last longer, and sometimes just as one joint settles down, another one flares up.

The urate crystals may also form in other tissues, such as fingers, hands, elbows, or ear lobes, and may be visible as white or yellow nodules called tophi (toe-fye). They can also form in the kidneys and produce kidney stones, which can cause severe pain as they pass from the kidney to the bladder.

Treatment of an acute gout attack is with anti-inflammatory drugs and pain killers. Once the attack has settled, treatment is aimed at reducing the frequency of future attacks. Often medication is given to reduce the amount of urate in the body so that it won't form crystals. Blood levels of uric acid are monitored to get the dose of medication right and to make sure it's continuing to work. Different treatments are available, so changes can be made if necessary.

Being overweight can bring on gout and make it more difficult to control, so getting down to a healthy weight is important. Certain foods, as well as alcohol, can raise the urate level in the body and make gout worse, so care must be taken to avoid these foods.

With effective treatment and regular monitoring, attacks can be kept to a minimum and long-term complications avoided.

Chapter 2

What is gout?

Gout is a form of arthritis affecting just a single joint or a small number of joints and is caused by crystals within the joint. Although various joints may be affected, the first joint of the big toe is most commonly involved. Symptoms include severe joint pain with swelling, tenderness, redness, and warmth. Sometimes there may be systemic symptoms such as fever, chills, and malaise. Doctors call these attacks acute gout or gout flares. Attacks occur up to several times a year. Typically, someone with a first attack of gout will have another within a year.

In between attacks, there are no symptoms, but gout crystals are slowly forming in joints and other tissues, ready to cause problems later. These periods are called intercritical gout.

As time goes by, attacks may affect more joints and last longer. A more chronic form eventually occurs in some people, with inflammation often moving from joint to joint or causing joint damage and persistent pain.

The crystals that cause gout may also cause problems away from the joints, collecting as nodules under the skin, called tophi (toe-fye), or collecting in the kidney, where they can cause kidney stones.

This third stage of gout, with persistent symptoms, tophi and progressive damage, doctors call chronic tophaceous gout. The time between the first attack and this stage of continuous gout symptoms varies, but on average, it takes about ten years.

Chapter 3

What causes gout?

Gout is caused by crystals in joints and sometimes in other tissues such as the fingers, ears, and kidneys.

The crystals are composed of a chemical called monosodium urate, or urate for short. As seen in Figure 11, the crystals are needle-shaped, so it's not hard to imagine why they cause pain in the joint. The immune system recognises them as abnormal, and this results in inflammation.

The problem occurs because urate is not very soluble. Suppose you produce too much urate or don't get rid of it quickly enough in the urine. In that case, it can build up to levels where there's just too much to remain dissolved in the blood and body fluids, so it begins to crystallise out. Salts are usually more soluble in warm water than in cold. It's for this reason, in gout, that these urate crystals are more commonly found in the cooler parts of the body, such as fingers, toes, and ear lobes.

The most common reason for having high levels of urate in the body is not getting rid of it quickly enough through the kidneys and into the urine. In some people, this may be due to inherited genetic factors that determine how well the kidney can excrete urate. People whose overall kidney function is reduced may also retain urate and other body waste products.

Some drugs can reduce the ability of the kidneys to excrete urate. The most common drugs to do this are the diuretics, or 'water tablets' used to treat high blood pressure and fluid retention by making the kidneys excrete more water. A particular family of diuretics, the thiazide diuretics are often singled out as being especially bad, but all diuretics can cause gout. Commonly prescribed diuretics are listed in the table below.

Commonly prescribed diuretics		
Amiloride	Chlorthiazide	Methylchlorthiazide
Bendroflumethiazide	Eplerenone	Metolozone
Brinzolamide	Furosemide	Torasemide
Bumetanide	Hydrochlorthiazide	Triamterene
Chlortalidone	Indapamide	Trichlormethiazide

Table 1: Commonly prescribed diuretics

Urate levels can also be raised if the body produces too much of it. In most cases, we cannot yet tell why certain people produce higher amounts of urate, but in some cases, the cause can be determined. In some of these cases, there are inherited genetic factors, often affecting certain enzymes involved in urate production. Obesity is another cause since urate production correlates with a person's body surface area – simply put, the 'rounder' you are, the bigger your surface area, and the more urate you produce.

Urate is produced by the breakdown of DNA and related molecules, so conditions that cause increased cell turnover can also cause raised urate levels and lead to gout. Such conditions include lymphoma, leukaemia, cancer treatment, and psoriasis.

The third reason that urate levels can be raised is from eating a lot of foods rich in a group of chemicals that get broken down by the body to produce urate. These chemicals are called purines. Foods rich in purines include offal (such as liver, kidneys and sweetbreads), consommé, meat gravies and broths, certain fish and shellfish (anchovies, herring, sardines, and mussels), and asparagus. We're sorry to tell you this, but a particularly rich source of purines is beer, including non-alcoholic beers.

Alcohol is, in fact, a particular villain in the case of gout, increasing urate levels in three ways. Firstly, it may stimulate urate production by the liver; secondly, it blocks the excretion of urate by the kidney; and thirdly, some beers contain quite a lot of purines – and we tend to drink quite large volumes of beer.

What are purines?

Purines are nitrogen-containing chemicals found widely in nature. They form key components of both DNA and RNA in the body. They are also essential for communication signals sent within and between cells.

Purines are found in high concentrations in meat and meat products, especially in internal organs such as liver and kidneys. Certain kinds of seafood are high in purines – examples are herring, mackerel and scallops, whilst most vegetables are low in purines – with a few exceptions such as lentils, black eye peas and spirulina.

Caffeine and theobromine (the stimulant chemical in tea) are both purines; however, consumption of tea and coffee does not increase urate levels in the blood; in fact, drinking coffee (but not tea) actually lowers urate levels and reduces the risk of gout. In studies carried out over many years, people who drank six or more cups of coffee had half the risk of developing gout as non-coffee drinkers.

More information about purines in the diet can be found on page 82.

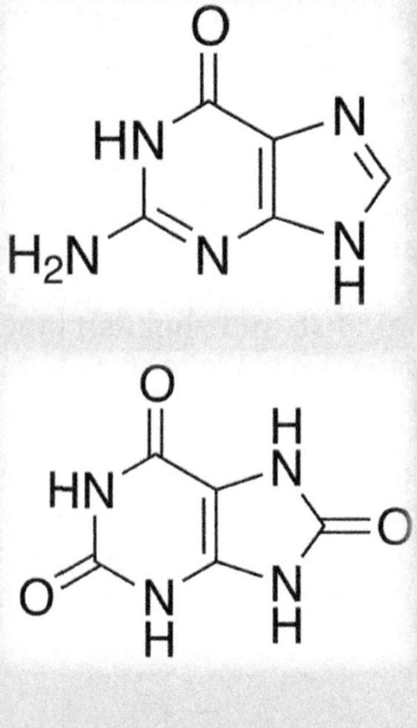

Figure 1: Structure of the purine guanine and of uric acid

The top molecule, the purine guanine, is one of the building blocks of DNA.

As you can see, the bottom molecule, uric acid, which is produced by the breakdown of guanine, is very similar.

Chapter 4

Who gets gout, and how common is it?

Gout is the most common form of arthritis caused by inflammation of the joints; three to four times more common than rheumatoid arthritis. The number of people affected varies from country to country, typically with more people having gout in wealthier countries. Within countries, gout is more common in poorer communities than in richer ones. Around 1.5% to 2.5% of people have gout in Western countries, equivalent to about 1 in 40 to 1 in 70 people. Hence, many people worldwide have gout: about 9.5 million in North America, 7.2 million in Europe, and an estimated 54 million worldwide. You can see more details on the number of people with gout in Table 2.

Men are affected with gout three times more often than women, so about three-quarters of people with gout are men. For example, that means that in the US, around 1 in 44 men and 1 in 133 women have gout. These are overall figures. If we just look at people middle-aged and above, these rates are a lot higher.

Each year, on average, one man in 1700 and 1 woman in 6000 will develop gout.

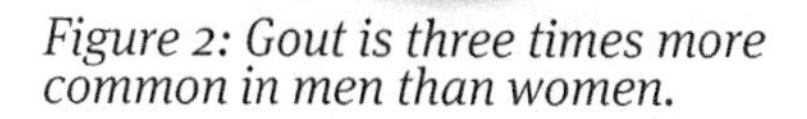

Figure 2: Gout is three times more common in men than women.

Country	How many people have gout			How many people get gout each year	
	Number	%	1 in ...	Number	1 in ...
Australia	542,462	2.4	1 in 42	65,421	1 in 2000
Canada	879,030	2.6	1 in 39	106,196	1 in 1667
France	681,794	1.1	1 in 91	85,058	1 in 3333
Germany	1,008,184	1.3	1 in 80	124,017	1 in 3333
Ireland	43,580	1.0	1 in 105	5661	1 in 5000
Italy	646,644	1.1	1 in 90	92,501	1 in 3333
New Zealand	106,210	2.5	1 in 39	13,921	1 in 2000
South Africa	284,099	0.5	1 in 189	56,883	1 in 5000
Spain	517,665	1.2	1 in 84	64,691	1 in 3333
UK	713,508	1.1	1 in 88	95,850	1 in 3333
USA	8,655,566	2.8	1 in 36	1,005,047	1 in 1667
Europe	7,198,610	0.9	1 in 112	1,090,583	1 in 5000
World	53,871,846	0.7	1 in 139	9,222,886	1 in 5000

Table 2: Number of people with gout in selected countries
(Source: Global Health Data Exchange – some sources have higher estimates, for example, some suggest that 3.9% of Americans have gout.)

In almost all countries the incidence of gout is rising. The cause is probably a mixture of ageing populations, the epidemic of obesity, and diets that are progressively higher in meat and processed foods. In the future, more and more people will be affected by gout.

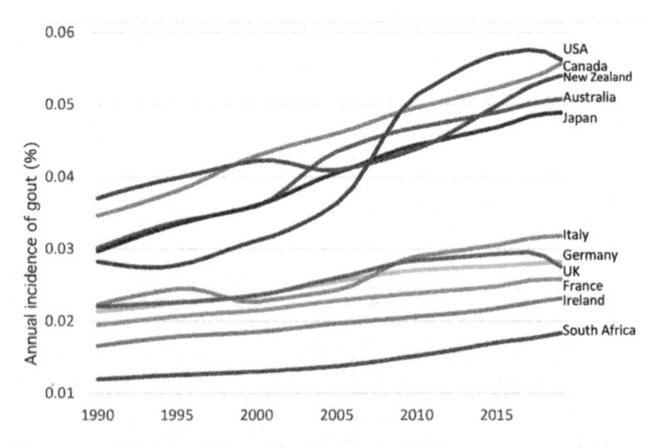

Figure 3: The incidence of gout is rising year on year
(Source: Global Health Data Exchange)

Ethnicity also plays a role in our likelihood of developing gout. African-American men are 1.6 times more likely to get gout than their white counterparts. Hmong Chinese men living in Minnesota have double the risk of gout compared to the general U.S. population. In New Zealand, Maori and Pacific Islanders have a 2 to 2.5 times higher rate of gout than New Zealanders of European ancestry.

The likelihood of having gout increases as we get older, so the typical gout patient is a man of middle age or older or a post-menopausal woman.

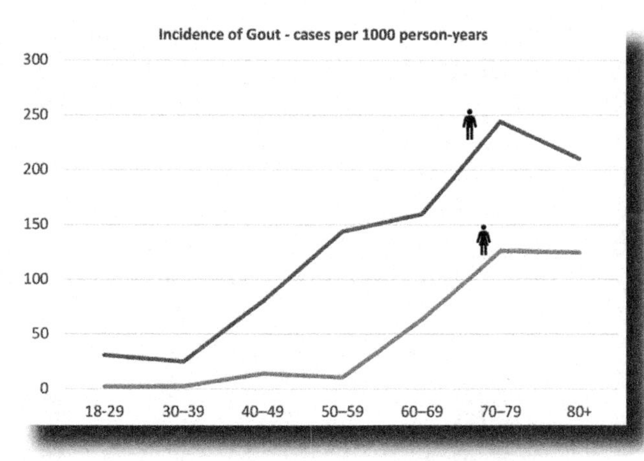

Figure 4: Gout becomes more common as we age

For some reason, gout attacks seem to occur more often in the spring, and then decline steadily over the year. In one study, gout attacks occurred almost 50% more often in spring compared to winter.

As we have already seen, gout is caused by urate crystals in joints and other tissues. It therefore makes sense that higher levels of urate in the blood lead to an increased risk of gout. While it is possible to have gout without raised blood uric acid levels and high uric acid levels but no gout, the risk of gout increases once your blood uric acid level rises above 6 mg/dL (0.36 mmol/L). At 8 mg/dL (0.48 mmol/L) the risk of gout has risen tenfold, and by 10 mg/dL (0.59 mmol/L) it is seventy times higher[1].

In some people, blood uric acid levels are high because of genetic factors they inherited from one or both parents. Many genes are associated with raised urate levels and the risk of gout. Though generally, these genes have only a small effect, several genes together can have a more significant effect. It has been estimated that genetic factors are responsible for between 45% and 73% of a person's urate level. This genetic effect is amplified by the behaviours we choose, such as what we eat and how much alcohol we drink.

Since urate is excreted from the body through the kidneys, it stands to reason that if the kidneys aren't working correctly, urate can build up in the body, and this can lead to gout. Consequently, people with chronic kidney disease have three times higher risk of gout.

So far, the factors we have discussed are beyond our control. Now let's move on to those we can control.

---

1 Whilst it is crystals of poorly soluble monosodium urate that cause gout, urate circulates in the blood as uric acid. The body's urate levels are assessed by measuring uric acid levels in the blood.

Certain foods rich in purines are broken down in the body to produce large amounts of urate. Eating a diet rich in such foods is likely to lead to higher urate levels and hence to a higher risk of gout. Such foods include meat, seafood, alcohol, and the sweetener high fructose corn syrup. From this observation comes the association of gout with historical royalty, who are popularly thought to have gorged on game and other rich foods. In contrast, those who eat a diet rich in fruit, vegetables, low-fat dairy and coffee have a lower risk of gout.

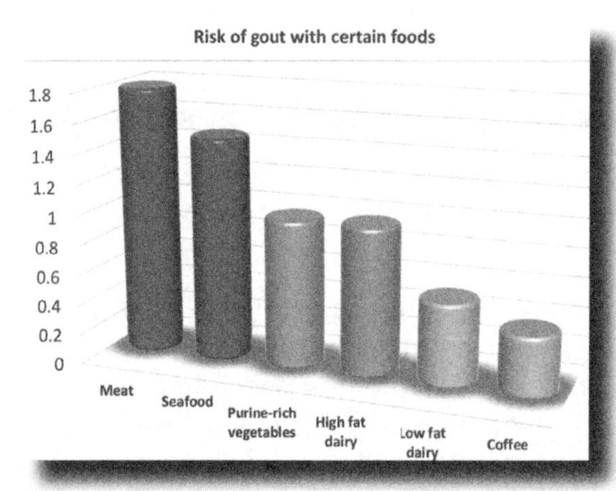

Figure 5: Different foods can increase or decrease the risk of gout

As Figure 5 shows, eating a lot of meat can almost double the risk of gout, whilst drinking lots of coffee more than halves the risk.

We will come back to look at how diet affects gout in much more detail later.

Alcohol consumption has a clear association with gout. Drinking lots of beer and spirits, but perhaps not wine, leads to a tripling of risk for gout, as shown in Figure 6. There's clearly a dose-response, where the more you drink, the higher your chance of getting gout. Beer is a rich source of dietary purines, and alcohol, in general, increases the production of urate by the liver and reduces the excretion of urate by the kidneys, thus raising the body's urate levels in three ways.

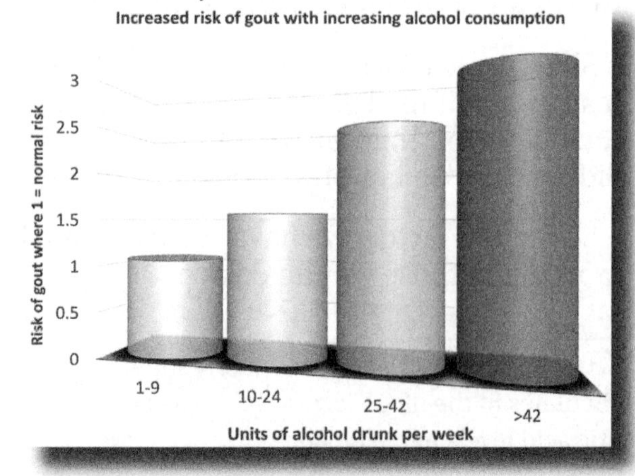

Figure 6: Drinking more alcohol increases the risk of gout.

(One unit is equivalent to a single measure of spirits, half a pint of beer, or two-thirds of a 125ml glass of wine.)

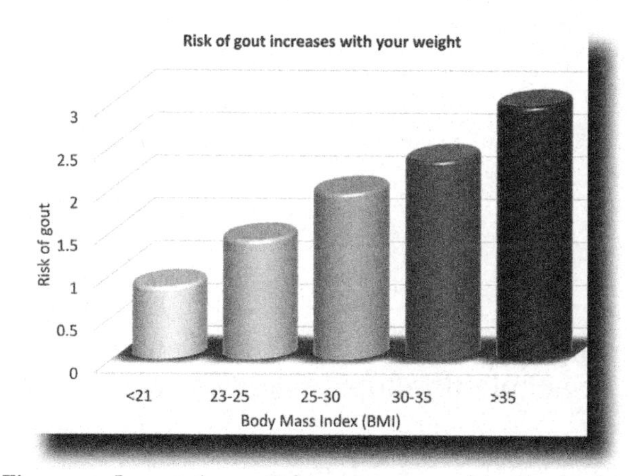

Figure 7: Increasing weight, as measured by the body mass index (BMI), increases gout risk.

Being overweight is another major risk factor for developing gout, and again there is a clear relationship between how overweight someone is and how much their risk of gout is increased. Someone with a BMI* of more than 35 has triple the risk of gout compared to someone of a 'healthy' weight.

To put that in context, if you're 5 ft 8 in tall, your BMI would be 35 if you weighed 229 pounds (16 st 5 lb). Or, if you prefer your measurements in metric: If you're 1 m 73 cm tall, your BMI would be 35 if you weighed 104 kg.

Certain medications increase the risk of gout. Particularly blameworthy in this respect are diuretics, so-called 'water tablets' used to treat high blood pressure or fluid retention – see Table 1 for a list of commonly prescribed diuretics. Diuretics increase blood uric acid levels by 6 to 21% by blocking its excretion by the kidneys. This rise in urate roughly doubles the risk of gout.

Low dose aspirin (≤ 325 mg/day), as used to prevent heart attacks or stroke, can also increase urate levels and increase the risk of gout. Interestingly, higher doses of aspirin increase the excretion of urate from the body. If you need aspirin to prevent a heart attack or stroke, the increased risk of gout can be negated by taking urate-lowering drugs such as allopurinol at the same time.

Less commonly used drugs that may also raise urate levels include the anti-TB drugs ethambutol and pyrazinamide, testosterone, the HIV drug didanosine, the immunosuppressant drugs cyclosporine and tacrolimus (both used to prevent rejection of transplanted organs), and cytotoxic chemotherapy drugs used to treat cancer.

* The BMI, or Body Mass Index is a measure that uses your height and weight to work out if your weight is healthy. A healthy BMI is 18.5 to 24.9. A BMI of 25 to 29.9 is classified as overweight, and a BMI of 30 or above is considered obese.

In summary

Gout is the most common form of arthritis caused by inflammation of the joints, and the number of people developing gout increases every year.

The risk factors for developing gout can be divided into three groups: those we have no control over, those we do have control over, and the third group are the medicines we take - so we have some control over these in collaboration with our doctors.

Things we cannot control	Things we can control	Medication
Male sex	Diet rich in purine containing foods	Diuretics
Middle age or older	Excessive intake of high fructose corn syrup	Low dose aspirin
Ethnicity	Alcohol intake > 9 units/week	Some anti-TB drugs
Blood uric acid level > 7.0 mg/dL (> 0.42 mmol/L)	Being overweight (BMI > 25)	Testosterone
Genetic factors		HIV drug didanosine
Chronic kidney disease		Immunosuppressants cyclosporine and tacrolimus
		Cytotoxic anti-cancer drugs

Chapter 5

How do I know if I have gout?

You should be suspicious that you may have gout if you develop a rapid onset of pain in a single joint, especially if it's the first joint of your big toe. Although the big toe is the most frequently affected joint, the instep, ankle, knee, wrist, and elbow are also commonly involved. Rarely gout may also affect the hip, pelvic, shoulder, collarbone, or neck joints. Gout affecting the first joint of the big toe is sometimes called podagra, an Old English word first mentioned in a 10th century Anglo-Saxon book of remedies.

The pain often begins at night and becomes more and more severe over a few hours, sometimes to the point of being excruciating. The affected joint may become swollen and very tender. The skin over the joint may be red or even purplish, often tight and shiny, and feel warm.

Sometimes the inflammation of the joints is accompanied by general symptoms of fever, chills, and general malaise.

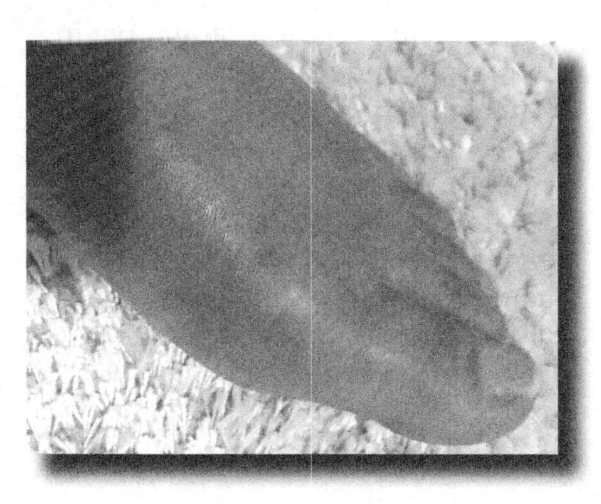

Figure 8: The first joint of the big toe is the joint most commonly affected by gout.

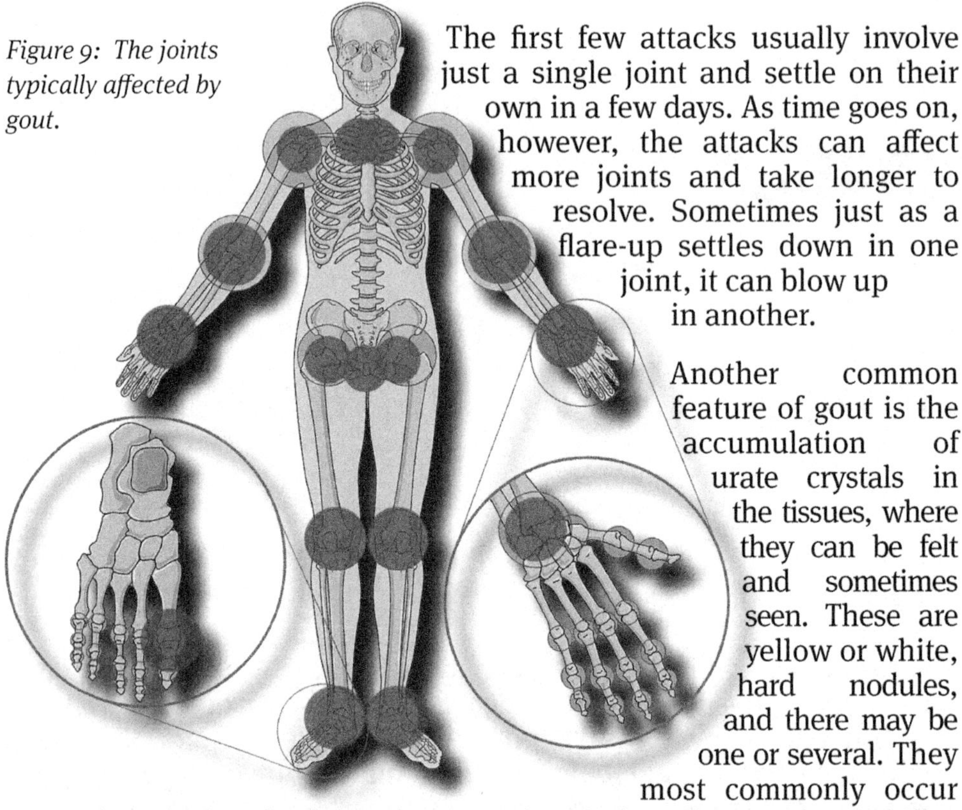

Figure 9: The joints typically affected by gout.

The first few attacks usually involve just a single joint and settle on their own in a few days. As time goes on, however, the attacks can affect more joints and take longer to resolve. Sometimes just as a flare-up settles down in one joint, it can blow up in another.

Another common feature of gout is the accumulation of urate crystals in the tissues, where they can be felt and sometimes seen. These are yellow or white, hard nodules, and there may be one or several. They most commonly occur in the fingers, hands, feet, the outside of the elbows, the Achilles tendons, and the earlobes. These nodules, called tophi (toe-fye), are usually painless but can sometimes become painful, particularly at the elbow. Occasionally they can break through the skin to reveal their chalky contents. If they occur within a joint, they can damage that joint.

Because urate crystals can also form in the kidneys, about one in five people with gout develop kidney stones. If these stones begin to move down the ureter from the kidney to the bladder, they can cause severe pain. Moving kidney stones typically cause intermittent, severe pain in the flank, kidney or genital regions, associated with nausea, vomiting, and sometimes blood in the urine.

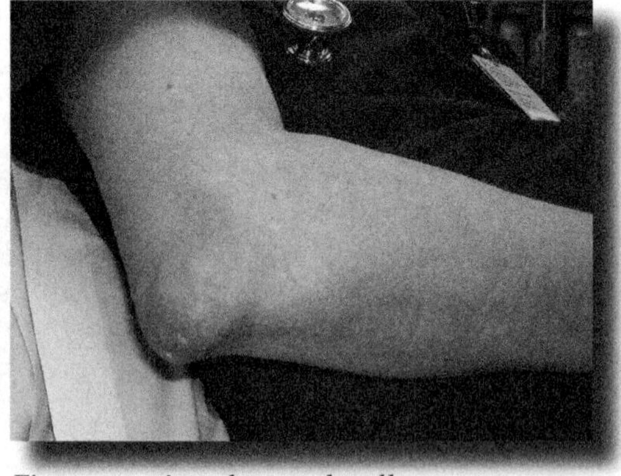

Figure 10: A tophus at the elbow.

Chapter 6

What other conditions can gout be confused with?

An attack of gout is quite characteristic. Indeed, once you've had one attack, you will recognise a future one. However, some other conditions can mimic gout or be similar enough to cause confusion. For this reason, it is essential to get a firm diagnosis from a doctor when the attacks first start rather than trying to diagnose yourself.

A perfect example of this is a bacterial joint infection. A joint infection can come on rapidly. The joint is red, swollen, and hot, and it can be very painful. In other words, it looks and feels just like gout. The difference is that while a gout flare-up will settle by itself in a few days, a joint infection will just go from bad to worse; the joint surfaces may become badly damaged, the bone itself may become infected, and the infection can get into the bloodstream and become life-threatening. The take-home message here should be very clear: a first attack of what appears to be gout needs to be checked out by a doctor.

Although an attack of gout may be associated with a fever, an inflamed joint together with a raised body temperature could also be a warning sign of infection in the joint or elsewhere, including serious infections such as an infected heart valve, rheumatic fever or Lyme Disease.

Another red flag for conditions that require urgent treatment is a sudden onset of joint pain in a young, sexually active individual. This can occur as a reaction to a sexually transmitted infection (usually Chlamydia or gonorrhoea) or direct spread of the infection via the bloodstream to the joint (gonorrhoea). There may be a current or recent rash, genital discharge, or a burning pain on passing urine, but these signs are not always present.

Urgent treatment should also be sought by anyone with a known bleeding disorder (such as haemophilia) or who is taking anticoagulants (such as warfarin or coumarin), as a sudden onset of pain and swelling in a joint could indicate bleeding into the joint.

A swollen, painful joint may also be the result of a recent injury. Usually, this is obvious, but occasionally the injury can go unnoticed.

Several rheumatological conditions may have similarities with gout. Rheumatoid arthritis usually affects multiple joints, which all flare up and then settle down together. Flare-ups tend to be more gradual in onset than gout. However, a rapid onset can sometimes occur, but episodes typically last longer than with gout.

However, there is a variant called palindromic rheumatism, which sometimes precedes the onset of rheumatoid arthritis, and which is very similar to gout. Usually, only one or a small number of joints are affected, and the pain can be just as severe as gout. Like gout, it also tends to settle down of its own accord in a few days.

Patients with the skin disease psoriasis can also get a form of arthritis called psoriatic arthropathy. Confusingly, they do not always have any signs of psoriasis on their skin. Typically, this affects the last joints of fingers or toes, though it can also affect larger joints and the lower back. The joint symptoms tend to be ongoing rather than occurring in discrete episodes like gout.

Osteoarthritis is caused by joint inflammation and damage to the joints from wear and tear, so it is common in older people and in younger people who put heavy stress on their joints, such as athletes. Joint symptoms in osteoarthritis tend to be very gradual in onset and are usually continuous rather than episodic. The pain is typically more of an ache than the severe pain of gout.

Sometimes rather than the joint itself, it's the structures around the joint, such as tendons and ligaments, that become inflamed. In this case, the joint itself is usually not tender. However, there may be localised tenderness just around the affected structure. Typically, the pain comes on when you move the joint yourself, but not if someone else moves the joint for you.

We discussed earlier the seriousness of a bacterial joint infection. A variety of other infections can cause joint symptoms as part of a broader illness. A reactive arthritis can be associated with certain sexually transmitted diseases (usually Chlamydia or gonorrhoea, as mentioned earlier) and also with gastrointestinal infections. One or several joints can be affected, and these are more commonly in the legs or toes. It usually affects joints symmetrically on both sides of the body. There may be an associated fever and a feeling of malaise.

Lyme Disease is a complex infection affecting many body systems, and an important diagnosis not to miss. Often there is a history of a tick bite, but these can easily go unnoticed. There tends to be aching in multiple joints early in the disease and later swelling and mild pain in larger joints, particularly the knees. There may be fever, malaise, general muscle aching, and a rash.

Some viral infections can cause joint inflammation, but this usually affects multiple joints and is characterised more by aching than the severe pain of gout.

Two uncommon conditions may cause joint pains in children and teenagers. Rheumatic fever usually follows a throat infection, causes joint pains in the wrists, elbows, ankles, and knees, and tends to move from joint to joint, lasting about two weeks in total. There is usually an associated fever. Juvenile idiopathic arthritis causes pain and swelling in multiple large and small joints, often associated with fever, rash, eye inflammation, swollen lymph glands, and other features. Confusion of either of these conditions with gout is unlikely as gout is rare in children and adolescents.

Finally, two other conditions, like gout, are associated with the deposition of crystals in joints and other tissues. In pseudogout, larger joints are usually affected, particularly the knees. Symptoms tend to be milder than in gout. People with pseudogout do not develop tophi. Basic calcium phosphate deposition disease can mimic gout, with rapid onset of pain and swelling together with a fever and feeling unwell. It may affect the big toe.

In summary

Signs	May be due to	Risk if not treated
A swollen, red, warm joint with a reduced range of movement	A bacterial joint infection	Permanent joint damage Spread of infection to bone or into the bloodstream
A painful joint with a fever	A bacterial joint infection	Permanent joint damage Spread of infection to bone or into the bloodstream
A painful joint with broken skin and signs of skin infection around the joint	A bacterial joint infection	Permanent joint damage Spread of infection to bone or into the bloodstream
Sudden onset joint pain in a young, sexually active person	Gonococcal arthritis	Permanent joint damage. Spread of infection to bone or into the bloodstream
New joint pain and swelling in a person with a bleeding disorder or who is taking anticoagulants	Bleeding into the joint	Permanent joint damage

Table 3: You should see a doctor straight away if you have any of these symptoms

Condition	Joint(s) affected	Other features
Gout	Most commonly, 1st joint of the big toe. Often instep, ankle, knee, wrist & elbow. Rarely hip, pelvic, shoulder, collarbone or neck joints. Usually just one joint. Later may involve several joints.	Rapid onset. Severe pain. Joint swollen, tender and hot. Skin over joint red/purple, tight and shiny. Sometimes fever, chills and malaise. Initially settles after 2-3 days. Later it may take longer to resolve. Tophi (nodules). Sometimes kidney stones.
Pseudogout	Mostly the knee, but sometimes the wrist, shoulder or ankle. May affect multiple joints	May occur in attacks like gout or may give continuing low-grade joint pains. Attacks tend to be less severe than gout.
Basic calcium phosphate crystal deposition disease	Shoulder most commonly affected. Less commonly hips, feet and hands.	Comes on over a few hours. Affected area swollen, tender, hot and red. Sometimes fever and mild malaise. Can mimic an acute gout attack of the big toe.
Palindromic rheumatism	Usually affects a single joint, occasionally several – most commonly knees and fingers.	Sudden onset joint pain. Pain can be as severe as gout. There may be a fever. Settles completely in a few days.

Condition	Joint(s) affected	Other features
Rheumatoid arthritis	Usually affects multiple joints, typically fingers and toes. Can also affect wrists, elbows, shoulders, hips, knees and ankles but can involve any joint.	Gradual onset of joint pain, swelling, tenderness, and early morning stiffness. There may be general fatigue, malaise, loss of appetite, generalised weakness, or fever. Episodes last longer than gout.
Psoriatic arthropathy	Most commonly end joint of fingers and toes but can affect most joints, including the lower back.	Usually, but not always, the rash of psoriasis will be present on the skin. Tends to be ongoing rather than episodic.
Osteoarthritis	Most commonly affects fingers and toes, spine, hips, and knees.	More common in older people. Slow onset. Joints are usually not tender or red. Tends to be ongoing rather than episodic. Pain typically less severe than gout. May be associated with nodules on fingers that can resemble tophi.
Fractures and sprains	Any joint.	Usually, but not always, a recent injury

Condition	Joint(s) affected	Other features
Bacterial joint infection (including gonococcal arthritis)	Usually a single joint. Most commonly, ankle, knee, hip, wrist, elbow or shoulder	Comes on over a few hours to a few days. Moderate to severe pain Joint swollen, tender and warm. Skin over the joint may be red. There may be a fever. There may be a rash or genital discharge with gonococcal arthritis
Reactive arthritis	May affect a single joint, a few joints or many. More common in knees, ankles, hips and toes. Joints affected are usually asymmetrical. Back pain sometimes occurs.	Usually follows 1 - 3 weeks after gastroenteritis or a sexually transmitted infection (usually Chlamydia). Joint pain mild to severe. Fever, fatigue and weight loss may occur. There may be pain in the sole of the foot and Achilles tendon, rashes, pain on passing urine and conjunctivitis.
Lyme disease	Early disease: Widespread aching joints. Late disease: One to a few large joints affected, especially knees.	May be a remembered tick bite. Early disease is a flu-like illness not easily confused with gout. Later there may be recurrent or persistent pain and swelling in affected joints. Pain not particularly severe.

Condition	Joint(s) affected	Other features
Bleeding into a joint	Usually affects a single joint.	Sudden onset of pain. May occur spontaneously or after injury. Mainly occurs in people with a known bleeding tendency such as haemophilia or on anticoagulant therapy.
Inflammation of tendons and other structures	Typically, larger joints such as shoulders, elbows, knees, hips, and wrists.	Pain is much worse when bending the joint yourself rather than if someone else moves the joint while you relax. May be tenderness over the inflamed structure though the joint itself is usually not tender.

Table 4: Conditions with which gout may be confused.

Chapter 7

When should I see a doctor?

As we have seen, although gout is a reasonably distinctive disease, almost all aspects of the condition can be mimicked by other conditions. Without having a laboratory identify the specific crystals from the joint, you cannot be entirely sure that you have gout. You may have a condition with serious consequences if left untreated or treated incorrectly. For this reason, you need to see a doctor if you have symptoms that you think may be due to gout.

Once a diagnosis of gout has been confirmed, you should plan with your doctor for how future flare-ups will be treated. Your doctor will probably give you some medication to keep on standby to begin taking if you have another attack. You will learn to recognize attacks of gout and manage them yourself.

Treatment is aimed at reducing the frequency of attacks. If you continue to have frequent attacks, you should see your doctor to find a more effective preventative strategy.

You should also see a doctor if you have an attack that is noticeably different from previous episodes. It could be something else.

Chapter 8

How will the doctor diagnose gout?

In a typical attack, particularly one affecting the big toe, the doctor can strongly suspect that the symptoms are due to gout. The presence of tophi (nodules) or previous similar attacks makes the diagnosis even more likely.

However, it is important to confirm the diagnosis and ensure that it's not something like a joint infection that could have severe consequences if not appropriately treated or a similar condition like pseudogout that may require different treatment. The diagnosis is confirmed by taking a little fluid from the affected joint for examination. This procedure, called joint aspiration, is done under sterile conditions to avoid introducing infection into the joint. A local anaesthetic injection or spray is used, and a small needle is used to collect fluid from the joint. Crystals can also be obtained from tophi.

If crystals are present in the joint fluid or tophi, these can be seen under the microscope. Different types of crystals have different shapes. Different crystals also bend the light in distinct ways when examined under polarized light through the microscope, giving them characteristic appearances. The monosodium urate crystals that cause gout look blue if they are horizontal and yellow if they are vertical, as shown in Figure 13.

Unless it is simply not possible, crystals should be obtained and examined in all new cases to make a cast-iron diagnosis of gout.

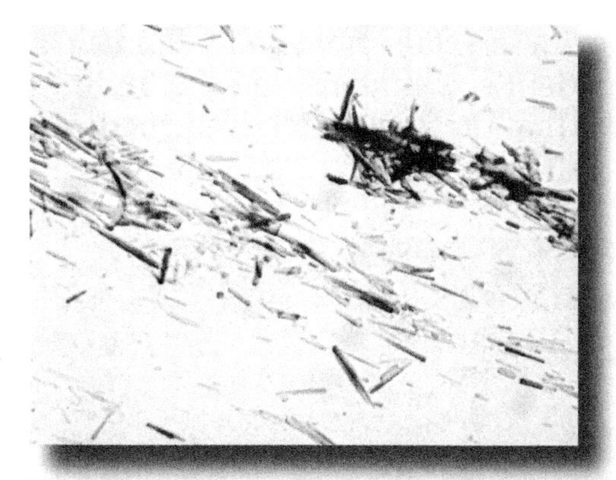

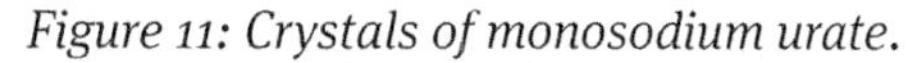

Figure 11: Crystals of monosodium urate.

The characteristic needle shape of gout's monosodium urate crystals is easy to see in this sample taken from a tophus.

It's not hard to imagine these sharp crystals causing pain when they're in a joint.

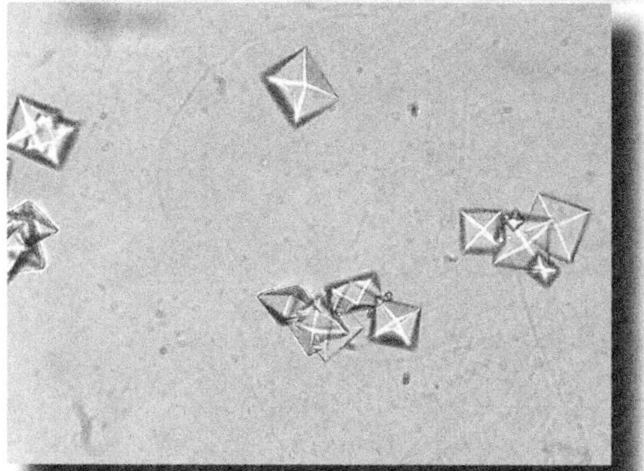

Figure 12: Crystals of calcium oxalate.

These crystals of calcium oxalate, which like monosodium urate can also cause arthritis, are clearly of a very different shape from those of uric acid.

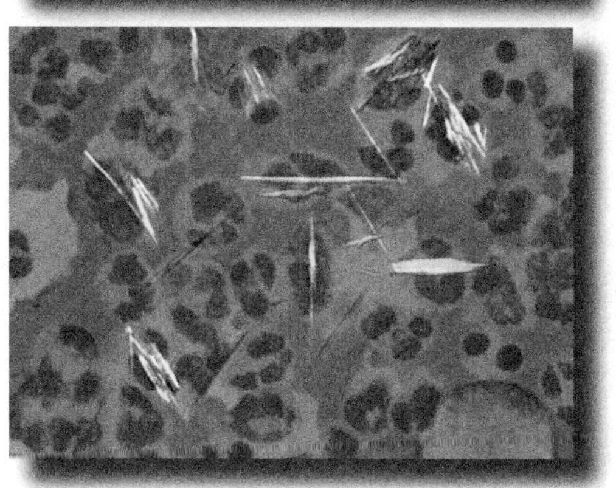

Figure 13: Crystals of uric acid under polarised light.

In case there is any confusion, the crystals can also be looked at under polarized light. Here you can see that monosodium urate crystals look blue when they lie horizontally and yellow when they are vertical.

As we have seen, it is vital to exclude a joint infection. With joint infections, white cells are present in large amounts in joint fluid, but they can be present in other causes of joint inflammation, including gout. For this reason, joint fluid is also studied in the lab to see if any bacteria are present.

The crystals you can see in Figure 13 were taken from a joint during a gout flare-up. In the background you can easily see the red and blue-stained white blood cells present in large numbers.

Where it is not possible to look for crystals from joint fluid or a tophus, doctors must rely on the patient's symptoms and the findings on examination. Studies have shown that these can effectively predict if someone has gout. See Figure 14.

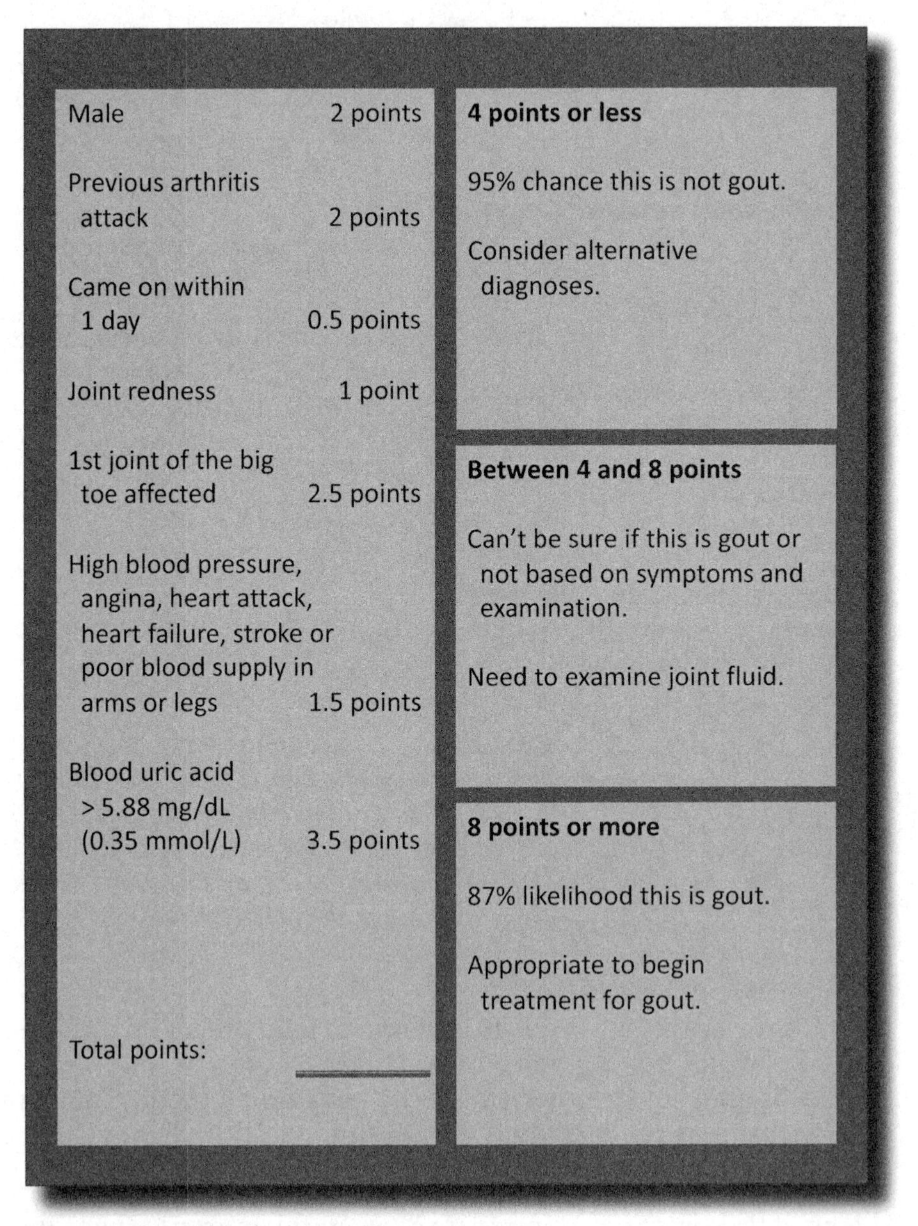

Figure 14: Algorithm for diagnosing gout

To use this chart, score the patient's characteristics using the attributes in the left column. Add up the total score and use the right column to interpret the score.

(From Keinhort, Janssens, Fransen & Janssen. Rheumatology 2015; 54:609-614)

The doctor will also measure levels of uric acid in the blood. A high level of uric acid is helpful to support a diagnosis of gout, but it is not enough on its own. Around one in three people with a proven gout attack have a normal blood uric acid level, and some people have a raised blood uric acid level but never get gout. This discrepancy means the blood uric acid level cannot prove that someone has gout or prove that they don't. Usually, the doctor will measure the blood uric acid level on two or three different occasions to understand an individual's baseline level. A 'normal' blood uric acid level is 2.5 - 8 mg/dL (0.15 - 0.47 mmol/L), but levels above 6 mg/dL (0.36 mmol/L) are high in the context of gout.

Sometimes the doctor will measure the amount of urate passed in the urine over 24 hours. The doctor or laboratory will give you a gallon container to do this. On waking in the morning, you empty your bladder into the toilet. After this, you collect all your urine in the container throughout the day and during the night. When you wake the next morning, you collect the first lot of urine you pass in the container. That is the end of the collection, and you should return the container to the doctor or laboratory.

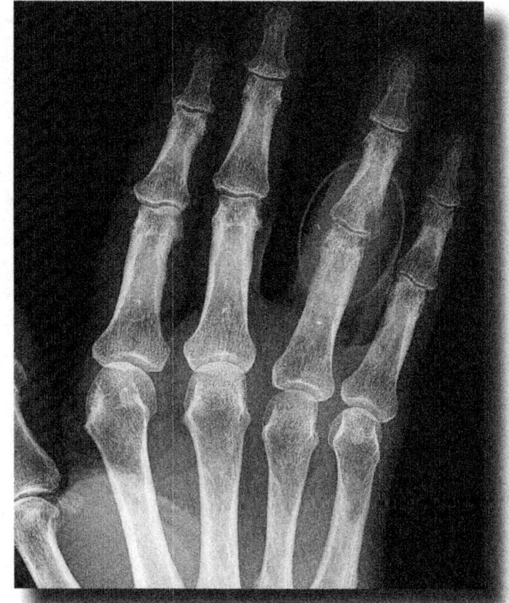

Figure 15: Note the punched out or gnawed area due to gout on the ring finger.

The amount of urate excreted in the urine over 24 hours may help the doctor work out if your gout is due to producing too much urate or not excreting enough. Normal 24-hour urine urate excretion is around 600 – 900 mg. If you excrete a lot less than this, the problem may be insufficient excretion of urate in the urine. If your level is significantly higher, it may be that you produce too much. Someone with a higher-than-normal urate excretion in the urine has an increased rate of developing kidney stones.

X-rays of the affected joints are sometimes taken, but they don't really add anything in a first attack of gout. The X-ray changes of gout take several years to develop. Eventually, damage to joints can be seen, as well as erosions of the small finger and toe bones that look as though they've been gnawed by a rat, as shown in Figure 15. Specialist technicians can often see urate crystals in joints on ultrasound, even in a first attack of gout. A particular type of CT scan, called DECT, is also good at seeing changes caused by gout.

To best manage gout going forward, your doctor will want to identify those risk factors which may have predisposed you to develop gout; these include chronic kidney disease, being overweight, specific medications that may increase the risk of gout, dietary factors, and any strong family history.

Gout often does not occur alone. Many people with gout have other medical conditions, so your doctor will want to investigate to see if you have any of these other conditions which also require attention. Conditions found commonly in people with gout include chronic kidney disease, being overweight – perhaps with resultant metabolic syndrome, high blood pressure, heart failure, diabetes, and abnormal lipids such as high cholesterol. In a review of more than 63,000 people with gout in the UK, one in four had cardiovascular disease, one in four had high blood pressure, and one in fourteen had diabetes. In a similar study in the US, three out of four people with gout (74%) had high blood pressure, more than four times higher than in similarly aged people without gout. A diagnosis of gout should be a wake up call to address other serious health issues.

In summary

It is vital to get a definitive diagnosis of gout. Other conditions can mimic gout, and some of these can have serious consequences if left untreated. You may potentially be embarking on life-long treatment, so you need to be certain the diagnosis is correct. The only way to be entirely sure is by finding urate crystals in fluid from an affected joint.

Other tests can support the diagnosis, such as the blood uric acid level and x-rays. Suppose joint fluid cannot be examined for some reason. In that case, the doctor will have to rely on these supporting factors and their own judgment and experience.

Once the diagnosis has been made, the doctor will look for risk factors that may have made you more likely to develop gout and also look for complications of gout and other conditions that frequently occur alongside gout and may also need treatment.

Definitive diagnosis	Finding urate crystals in joint fluid	
Supporting evidence	**Risk factors**	**Complications and co-existent conditions**
Blood uric acid level	Being overweight	Kidney stones
Amount of urate passed in the urine in one day	Family history of gout	High blood pressure
Joint x-rays	Chronic kidney disease	Cardiovascular disease
Joint ultrasound	Diet	Diabetes
DECT scans	Medications	Abnormal lipids
		Metabolic syndrome

Chapter 9

How is gout treated?

There are two aspects to the treatment of gout:

1. Treatment of an acute attack
2. Lowering blood uric acid levels and removing urate from the body to reduce the risk of future attacks and to get rid of tophi

We will look at both of these in some detail.

Note: More detailed information about the drugs used to treat gout can be found in Chapter 13.

Treatment of an acute gout attack

An attack of gout will settle down on its own in a few days, but because it can be excruciating, most people want some kind of treatment.

Starting treatment as early as possible means that the attack will settle more quickly. It is good practice to have a course of treatment on hand to be started at the first signs of an attack.

Most people are treated with one of the following medicines:

- A non-steroidal anti-inflammatory drug
- Colchicine
- A steroid – by mouth, by injection, or into the affected joint

These medicines are all equally effective. Which one to use comes down to the personal preference of patient and doctor, and sometimes which treatments are ruled out by other medical conditions or medicines being taken.

Attacks are most often treated with a **non-steroidal anti-inflammatory drug (NSAID)**. These are drugs such as naproxen, indomethacin, and ibuprofen, and they are usually effective. Pain relief is generally felt in a few hours, and over the next few days, they also reduce the inflammation in the joint.

Although NSAIDs are widely used and generally don't cause any problems, they can cause side effects. The most common unwanted effects are gastro-intestinal inflammation or bleeding, fluid retention, and effects on the kidney. They may also increase the risk of a heart attack. The elderly, people with previous stomach ulcers or indigestion, people taking anticoagulants (blood thinners), those with impaired kidney function, and people who are dehydrated are at higher risk of side effects. The minimum dose that treats the symptoms should be used. You should not take more than one NSAID at a time as the combination significantly increases the risk of side effects. NSAIDs are found in many over the counter medicines, so check with a doctor or pharmacist if in doubt. The exception is low dose aspirin being taken to prevent a heart attack or stroke. In this case, the aspirin should be continued. NSAIDs should be taken with food to protect the stomach lining and swallowed with at least a cup of water to ensure the tablets or capsules pass all the way to the stomach.

Because of these potential side effects, NSAIDs should be avoided if you:

- Have an active stomach or duodenal ulcer
- Have recurrent gastro-intestinal bleeding
- Are taking anticoagulants (blood thinners)
- Have moderate to severe kidney impairment
- Have cardiovascular disease, especially hard to control heart failure or high blood pressure
- Have had asthma or wheezing when taking NSAIDs before, including aspirin

There are many different NSAIDs on the market. Table 5 lists the most commonly used ones. Naproxen or indomethacin tend to be the first choices for gout.

Name	Usual dose Note that you may need a different dose. These 'standard' doses are provided only for general information. You need to talk to your doctor about the correct dose for you.	Maximum recommended daily dose
Celecoxib	100 mg or 200 mg once or twice daily	800 mg
Diclofenac	75 mg twice daily, or 50 mg three times daily, or 100 mg slow release once daily	150 mg
Etodolac	300 mg two or three times a day, or 400-500 mg twice daily	1200 mg
Fenoprofen	800 mg every six hours, reducing the dose quickly when the attack starts to settle	3200 mg
Flurbiprofen	100 mg two or three times daily	300 mg
Ibuprofen	400-800 mg three or four times daily	3200 mg
Indomethacin	50 mg three times daily until the pain begins to settle, then reduce the dose.	200 mg
Ketoprofen	100 mg three times daily	300 mg
Meclofenamate	50 mg three or four times daily	400 mg
Meloxicam	7.5 mg once daily	15 mg
Nabumetone	1000 mg once daily, or 500 mg twice daily	2000 mg
Naproxen	750 mg to begin, then 250 mg every eight hours	1500 mg
Oxaprozin	1200 mg once daily	1800 mg
Piroxicam	20 mg once daily	20 mg
Sulindac	200 mg twice daily	400 mg
Tiaprofenic acid	300 mg twice daily	600 mg
Tolmetin	400 mg three times daily	1800 mg

Table 5: Non-steroidal inflammatory drugs (NSAIDs) that may be used to treat gout.

An alternative to NSAIDs is **colchicine**, a traditional treatment made from the autumn crocus plant. If started within the first 12 to 24 hours of an attack, it can have a dramatic effect. It is much less effective if started more than 36 hours after the onset of an attack. Pain relief usually begins in 12 to 24 hours.

Colchicine is taken as an initial dose of 1 mg or 1.2 mg (depending on where you live, since different countries have different tablet strengths), followed by 0.5 mg or 0.6 mg one hour later. After that, 0.5 mg or 0.6 mg is taken once a day.

The most common side effects of colchicine are gastro-intestinal: nausea, vomiting, abdominal pain, and diarrhoea. In the past high doses of colchicine were used. With these doses almost everyone developed abdominal pains and diarrhoea, usually before they had any relief from their joint pain. As a result, many people are wary of taking colchicine. Today's low dose regimens are much less likely to cause side-effects, but some doctors haven't updated their prescribing practices and still use the old regimens.

The main reason why someone may not be able to take colchicine is if they are taking other medicines that stop the liver from breaking down colchicine. The drugs that do this the most are the HIV protease inhibitors (such as ritonavir, indinavir, lopinavir, dolutegravir, tipranavir and others), certain antifungals (such as fluconazole, voriconazole, ketoconazole and posaconazole), and the antibiotics clarithromycin and telithromycin. Taking any of these medicines at the same time as colchicine can lead to a build-up of dangerously high colchicine levels in the body. Interestingly, grapefruit juice has the same effect, so don't drink it when taking colchicine.

Colchicine is also effective at preventing future attacks and so may be continued after the attack has settled. People who have a gout attack while taking colchicine for prevention can still use it to treat the attack by briefly increasing the dose. Recommendations vary, so you need to talk to your doctor about what to take if you have an attack.

The third main alternative for treating a gout attack are **steroids**, or more precisely, corticosteroids. These can be taken as tablets (usually as prednisolone or prednisone) or given by injection into a muscle or into the affected joint itself.

Short courses of steroids do not usually cause problems for most people. They may cause mood changes or sleep disturbances, and they can increase blood sugar in people with diabetes.

Anyone with an ongoing infection should not be treated with steroids as they can suppress the immune system. Steroids also slow healing, so anyone with recent surgery and an unhealed wound should avoid steroids. Steroids can raise blood sugar, so people with poorly controlled diabetes are not usually treated with steroids.

For the rare individual who cannot be treated with NSAIDs, colchicine, or steroids, or who fail to get better with them, there are two new treatments that help block the inflammation caused by gout. These medicines, **anakinra** and **canakinumab**, must be given by injection and are primarily used in specialist centres.

Whichever medicine is used, treatment is continued for two or three days after the joint symptoms have settled to reduce the risks of it flaring up again. Typically, treatment will be taken for five to seven days.

In addition to the medication described here, the affected joint should be rested, and ice packs applied. Sometimes immobilizing the joint with a splint helps with the pain, as do bed cradles to keep the weight of bedclothes off inflamed toes.

Name	Usual dose
Colchicine	1 or 1.2 mg immediately, followed by 0.5 or 0.6 mg one hour later, then one or two 0.5 mg or 0.6 mg tablets daily.
Prednisone/Prednisolone	30 to 40 mg once daily
Anakinra	100 mg by injection once daily
Canakinumab	150 mg by injection as a single dose

Table 6: Non-NSAIDs used to treat an acute attack of gout

Prevention of future attacks

The frequency of recurrent attacks can be reduced through two strategies used alone or in combination:

1. Taking an anti-inflammatory like colchicine or NSAIDs.
2. Taking medication to reduce the amount of urate in the body

Colchicine is usually taken as 0.6 or 1.2 mg once daily (or 0.5 or 1 mg daily depending on which tablets are available in your country). If a flare-up begins whilst on this maintenance dose, an extra 1.2mg dose may be taken to abort the attack. However, if an extra 1.2mg dose has been taken in the past two weeks to treat an earlier flare-up, NSAIDs should be used rather than another extra dose of colchicine. Talk to your doctor to be clear on what they recommend for you.

When **NSAIDs** are used to prevent gout attacks, they are usually taken at a lower dose than those used to treat an acute attack to reduce the risk of side effects with long-term use.

Lowering the blood uric acid level and removing urate from the body to get rid of tophi and reduce the risk of future attacks

As we have seen, the number and frequency of attacks can be reduced with colchicine or non-steroidal anti-inflammatory drugs. Still, the urate crystals that remain in the body can cause progressive damage. Ideally, doctors aim to reduce the amount of urate in the body. Eventually, the tophi in the soft tissues and joints will dissolve and disappear.

Not everyone who has had an attack of gout needs to have their urate level reduced. Generally, this long-term treatment is given to individuals who:

- Have two or more gout attacks per year
- Have tophi in soft tissue or joints
- Have evidence of joint damage on X rays or scans
- Have kidney stones or chronic kidney impairment
- Have other medical conditions which prevent them from taking drugs usually used to treat or prevent gout

The amount of urate in the body can be reduced by:

- Blocking the production of urate
- Increasing the excretion of urate in the urine

The relationship between blood uric acid levels and gout attacks is a strange one. You can have a gout attack with a normal blood uric acid level, and you can have a high uric acid level and never get gout. Here's another strange fact: you can get an attack of gout when your uric acid level goes down, as well as when it goes up. In fact, it more commonly occurs when the uric acid level goes down.

As a result, there has been much debate about whether to start medication to reduce the urate level during an attack or wait until a few weeks after it has settled. Many doctors believe it is better to wait, but there is little evidence to support this. In fact, a recent study showed that starting urate lowering treatment during an attack did not make the attack last longer, and there was no increased risk of a further attack soon afterwards. Recent recommendations are to start urate-lowering treatment as soon as possible.

Since an attack is more likely to occur as the urate level falls, preventative therapy with colchicine or NSAIDs is given for the first three to six months of treatment to reduce urate.

A "normal" blood uric acid level, is 2.5 - 8 mg/dL or 0.15 - 0.47 mmol/L, depending on which units the laboratory uses. For someone with gout, the aim is to get the uric acid level to around the middle of this range.

For someone with gout but without tophi (urate nodules), treatment aims to get the uric acid level below 6 mg/dL (0.36 mmol/L). A lower level is desirable for someone with tophi as the tophi will dissolve and disappear. The blood uric acid level should be kept below 5 mg/dL (0.30 mmol/L) in these cases. It can take many months or even years for the tophi to disappear completely.

Blocking the production of urate

The drug most used to block urate production is **allopurinol**. It is usually started at a low dose (typically 100 mg) which is then increased until the blood uric acid reaches an appropriate level. Mild gastro-intestinal upsets are the most common side effects. However, allopurinol should be stopped if a rash develops. A rash can be a warning sign of a serious reaction that can lead to severe rashes and inflammation of the liver and other tissues. Certain ethnic groups, including people with Han Chinese, Korean and Thai ancestry, are at a higher risk of this reaction. For such people, it may be advisable to take a screening test for the genetic marker of this hypersensitivity (HLA-B*5801) before starting treatment with allopurinol.

For patients who can't take allopurinol or in whom allopurinol doesn't reduce uric acid levels enough, an alternative is **febuxostat**. Febuxostat works in the same way as allopurinol. One of the reasons people might stop taking allopurinol is if they develop a severe skin reaction. Unfortunately, the same can happen with febuxostat, and people who have had a reaction with allopurinol are at a higher risk of a similar reaction with febuxostat.

Febuxostat is started at a dose of 40 mg once a day which can be increased to 80 mg once a day after a few weeks if blood uric acid levels have not fallen enough.

In studies, people taking febuxostat had a higher risk of sudden death from cardiovascular causes such as heart attacks than people taking allopurinol. For this reason, febuxostat is reserved for people who can't take allopurinol or for whom allopurinol hasn't worked. Anyone who has cardiovascular disease should probably not take febuxostat.

For the few people on allopurinol or febuxostat whose blood uric acid level remains above 6 mg/dL (0.36 mmol/L) and who have at least two gout attacks per year or tophi that are not getting smaller, there is a third option, pegloticase.

Pegloticase is a version of the enzyme uricase, which breaks down uric acid. Most mammals have this enzyme, but most higher primates, including humans, don't. Pegloticase is effective at removing urate from the body. However, it must be given intravenously every two weeks, and it has a higher risk of side-effects that can be serious, notably a severe allergic reaction. It can also cause anaemia in people with an enzyme deficiency (G-6-PD deficiency) common in people with Mediterranean, African and Asian ancestry, who should be screened for this before starting pegloticase. Because it must be given by infusion, the risk of serious reactions and its high cost, pegloticase is mainly used only in specialist centres.

Increasing the excretion of urate in the urine

Another way to reduce urate levels in the body is by boosting its excretion in the urine with probenecid, sulphinpyrazone or lesinurad. Increasing urate excretion may be combined with blocking urate production as described above.

Urate crystals can form in the kidneys, causing kidney stones. Increasing the amount of urate in the urine increases this risk, so this kind of treatment is not used for individuals who already have kidney stones. Anyone taking this kind of medication needs to drink at least 3 litres / 6 pints of fluid each day to dilute the urate in the urine so that it won't form stones.

The drug most commonly used to increase urate excretion by the kidneys is **probenecid**. After an initial starting dose of 250 mg twice a day, blood uric acid levels are measured, and the dose of probenecid is increased as required. Side effects of probenecid include headache, nausea, loss of appetite and vomiting. Probenecid blocks the excretion of many drugs by the kidney, including NSAIDs, which can lead to toxicity. Therefore, you must talk to your doctor about all your medications before starting probenecid.

Sulphinpyrazone is an alternative to probenecid. It is more potent at increasing urate excretion, but it tends to cause more side effects. Common side effects include lower back pain and painful urination. Less commonly, people on sulphinpyrazone have reported severe allergic reactions, shortness of breath and gastrointestinal irritation.

A third drug, **lesinurad**, has recently been licenced in the US, and other countries are considering making it available. It works in the same way as probenecid but doesn't interact as much with other medicines making it more straightforward to prescribe for people on other drugs. In clinical studies, lesinurad caused kidney problems in some people. This was more common in people taking lesinurad alone. For this reason, it is added to allopurinol or febuxostat in people whose urate cannot be controlled with allopurinol or febuxostat alone.

When a urate-lowering medicine is first prescribed, the blood uric acid level is usually tested before starting medication and then every month. Using these results, the doctor will adjust the dose of medicine to the most effective level. Once stable, it is generally checked every six months.

Whichever medicine is chosen to lower urate levels in the body, it should be continued indefinitely.

Name	Usual dose
Allopurinol	Starting dose 50-100 mg once daily. May be increased up to 400 mg twice daily. Typical dose 300 mg once daily.
Febuxostat	Starting dose 40 mg once daily. May be increased to 80 mg once daily.
Pegloticase	8 mg by 2-hour infusion every two weeks

Table 7: Drugs used to block the production of urate

Name	Usual dose
Probenecid	250 mg twice daily. May be increased up to 500 mg four times daily.
Sulphinpyrazone	100 - 200 mg twice daily. May be increased up to 200 mg four times daily.
Lesinurad	200 mg once a day. Always given in combination with either allopurinol or febuxostat.

Table 8: Drugs used to increase the excretion of urate in the urine

In summary

In an acute attack of gout, anti-inflammatory medicines are used to stop the pain and inflammation as quickly as possible.

After the acute attack is over, the priority is to prevent future episodes. Anti-inflammatory drugs can do this and are usually continued for several months. Future attacks and complications can be reduced by lowering the amount of urate in the body.

The amount of urate in the body is usually reduced by blocking its production, but it can also be done by helping the body get rid of more urate through the kidneys and out in the urine.

The medicines used for each of these steps are given in the diagram below.

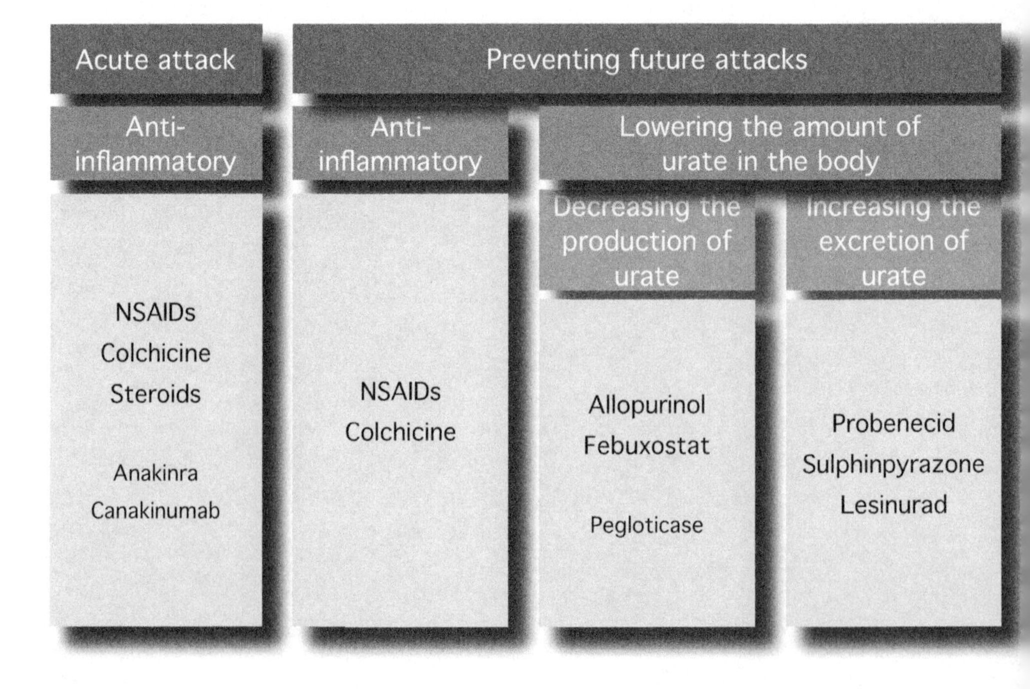

Chapter 10

What questions should I ask the doctor about my diagnosis and initial treatment?

This book aims to provide you with information and understanding so that you can talk with confidence to your doctor and understand the decisions they make. The question suggested here are meant as openings for discussion so that you can understand and be involved in the decisions made about your health. To participate in those discussions, you should have read the appropriate sections in the Handbook.

Ask about making a rock-solid diagnosis by examining joint fluid:

It is strongly recommended to be certain of the diagnosis by examining fluid from an inflamed joint or a tophus. In one study, more than half the people being treated for gout didn't have it! Your doctor may feel confident to diagnose gout simply from your symptoms. In such circumstances, it would be reasonable to ask: "What reassures you that it's gout rather than a joint infection or another type of crystal in the joint? Do you think examining the joint fluid would be useful?" (Chapter 8 on page 24)

Ask about preventing future attacks:

If you are visiting the doctor with an attack of gout for the first time, the priority is to treat the current symptoms. But it is also the time to start thinking about reducing the risk of future attacks. In the past, doctors were told to wait until an attack had resolved before starting urate-lowering medication. It was believed that starting such medication during an attack could prolong it. This now seems to be incorrect, and recent recommendations have been to begin urate-lowering treatment as soon as possible. You might want to ask your doctor, "I heard that reducing high uric acid levels in the blood can prevent future attacks and long-term complications. When do you plan to check my levels and decide whether to start me on urate-lowering treatment?"

Ask about your medications:

Any time a doctor writes you a prescription, you should ask: "Please would you explain what medication you are prescribing and what it's for." After listening carefully to the answer, you should ask: "Is there anything I need to know about this medication?" Tell the doctor about any other medical conditions you have, particularly liver, kidney and heart disease, as many of these will influence the decision of which medicine is right for you. Be sure to also tell your doctor about all the other medications you are taking, including over the counter medicines, herbal treatments and supplements, in case one of them might react badly with the drug you are being prescribed.

Chapter 11

What are tophi and how are they treated?

A tophus (toe-fuss) is a nodule caused by an accumulation of urate crystals in tissue. The plural is tophi (toe-fye). The name comes from the Latin word for loose, porous rock.

Because urate is less soluble at cooler temperatures, tophi tend to form in cooler parts of the body: fingers, hands, elbows, feet, Achilles's tendons, and ear lobes. If they are in the skin, or close to the skin, they can be felt, and may be seen as white or yellowish nodules.

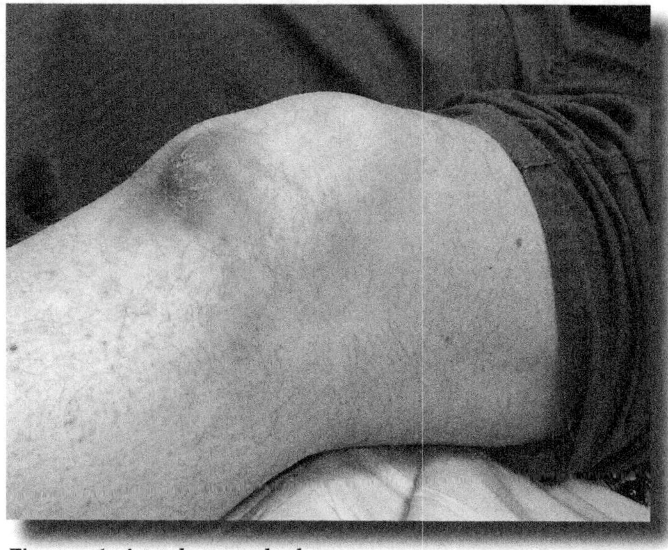

Figure 16: A tophus on the knee.

If a tophus is injured, the urate crystals within it can cause inflammation leading to pain, swelling and redness. This is seen most commonly at the elbow. A tophus may break through the skin, revealing its chalky contents.

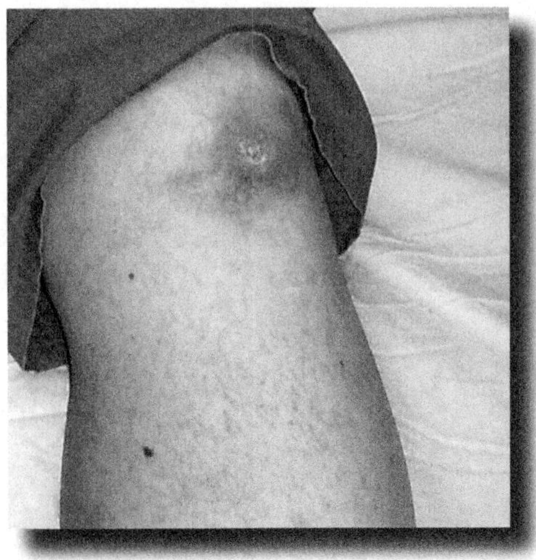

Figure 17: A tophus at the elbow

Tophi can also form in joints. Here they can damage the joint surfaces leading to typical arthritis pain, restricted movement at the joint, and possibly joint deformity.

Tophi are treated by reducing the body's urate level and keeping it low, as described in Chapter 9, and by maintaining good hydration (3 litres/6 pints of fluids a day.) Everyone with tophi should receive urate-lowering treatment. Over a period of months, the tophi slowly dissolve, get smaller, and disappear.

Occasionally, tophi can be removed surgically if they are particularly unsightly or inconvenient, or if they are causing problems, for example, by pressing on a nerve.

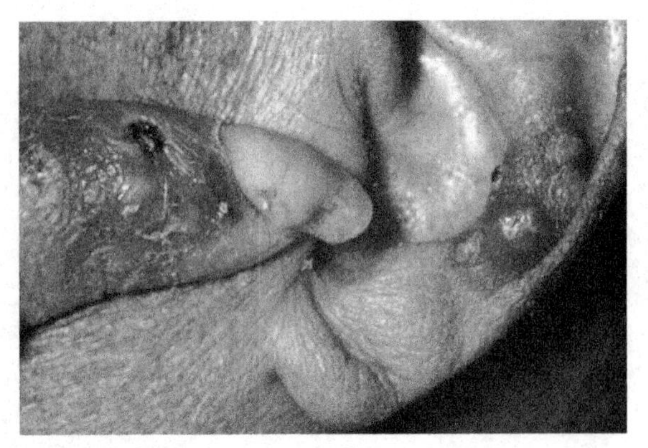

Figure 18: Tophi on the earlobe and finger.

Chapter 12

Can't I just rely on my doctor to choose the best treatment for me?

We are used to relying on our doctors to make the best decisions for our medical treatment. Unfortunately, doctors are overworked, the number of diseases they are supposed to know about is vast, and huge amounts of new information come out all the time. As a result, the standard of care patients receive is not always optimal. Gout has been described as one of the worst treated chronic diseases.

If you read the chapter, "How is Gout Treated?" you will have an idea of what good gout treatment looks like. Let's now look at what happens in the real world.

To be absolutely sure the diagnosis of gout is correct, crystals should be identified in fluid from a joint or tophus. In reality, less than 10% of people have joint fluid examined, so a diagnosis of gout may be missed or, more likely, made incorrectly. In a UK study of more than 63,000 people diagnosed with gout, more than half (57%) of the people taking allopurinol didn't actually have gout.

Most people with gout will meet the criteria for starting long-term urate-lowering treatment with allopurinol or similar. Yet, in a review of more than 115,000 people with gout in the UK, only a little over 1 in 3 (38%) were taking a urate-lowering medicine. Of those recently diagnosed with gout, only 19% were prescribed a urate-lowering medication within six months, and just 27% a year after being diagnosed. All the time their urate level is left elevated, crystals are being deposited in joints and kidneys and forming tophi, storing up problems for the future.

Allopurinol should be started at a low dose and then increased at monthly intervals until the blood uric acid reaches target levels. In a US study, only 20% of people on allopurinol ever reached their target uric acid level. Another 20% didn't achieve their target level, and fully 60% never had their uric acid level measured!

Doctors can also get confused about what the target level should be. Often, they will use the 'normal range' set by their local laboratory: the numbers reported with every blood test. My textbook here says that the normal range for uric acid is 1.5 to 8 mg/dL (0.09 to 0.48 mmol/L). But we know that the target uric acid level for someone with gout is less than 6 mg/dL (0.36 mmol/L), and for someone with tophi, it's less than 5 mg/dL (0.3 mmol/L). A doctor going by the lab's normal range could be happy with a uric acid level of 8 mg/dL, which would be terrible for someone with gout.

Between the lack of regular blood tests and confusion about the target levels, it is estimated that two-thirds of people with gout never reach their target uric acid levels. The consequences of this are needless gout attacks and, in the long term, tophi, joint damage, kidney stones and kidney damage.

When allopurinol is prescribed, very often, the dose is incorrect. Many doctors will simply prescribe what they think is a 'standard' dose rather than adjusting it based on blood uric acid levels. Most often, this results in the patient getting too low of a dose. In one review, the average dose of allopurinol taken by patients who reached their target uric acid level was 370 mg/day, yet overall, 97% of patients received a dose of 300 mg or less, far below the effective dose. It's little wonder that most people never reach their target uric acid level.

Although most people don't get a high enough allopurinol dose, some people get too much. People with poorly functioning kidneys often need a lower dose. In one review, more than 1 in 5 such patients (22%) were taking an amount higher than recommended for their degree of kidney disease. In another study, 1 in 4 (26%) were getting too high a dose.

As you know from the last chapter, when allopurinol is started and urate levels begin to fall, people often have a gout attack. Allopurinol should be started at a low dose and slowly increased to prevent attacks. At the same time, a preventative treatment with either a non-steroidal anti-inflammatory drug or colchicine should be given for the first 3 to 6 months to prevent attacks. In one review, less than half the people (48%) were prescribed an NSAID or colchicine; in another study, that figure was 42%, and in a third review, it was just 1 in 4 (26%). Not surprisingly, lots of people get gout attacks after starting allopurinol.

The problems aren't confined to allopurinol either; we just used these as an example. It's the same for other medicines: 1 in 3 people treated with colchicine don't get the recommended six-monthly blood tests to check for damage to the kidneys or bone marrow. One in 3 people with kidney impairment were receiving too high a dose of colchicine, with a risk of severe toxicity. Two-fifths of people on probenecid never had blood tests for their kidney function, even though these are important to avoid kidney damage. It goes on and on.

Clearly, just getting the correct dose prescribed by the doctor can be quite a challenge. Next, we must look at what people then do with their prescriptions. It turns out people tend not to take their medication very well. In one study, almost 3 out of 4 people (72%) were taking less than 80% of their prescribed allopurinol, either by taking a lower dose or missing doses. In another study, only 4 in 10 people were taking their urate-lowering medication properly. Another 4 in 10 were taking it on and off, and 2 in 10 weren't taking it at all. This is quite common for medicines with no apparent immediate benefit from taking them. You know if you miss a dose of pain killer for an agonizing toe, but you don't feel any difference if you miss your allopurinol dose, so it doesn't seem so important. Also, if people aren't given a preventative medicine for the first few months of urate-lowering treatment (which, as we've seen, happens to at least half), they may get one or more gout attacks, and this can lead to an incorrect belief that the treatment isn't working.

If you're not worried after reading this, you might like to go back and reread it because it's very concerning. The vast majority of people with gout are not getting treated correctly and, in consequence, are getting a lot sicker than they need to. It's not just about suffering unnecessarily with your gout either. In a US study of half a million people, those who received sub-optimal treatment for their gout had a 24% higher mortality – from any cause. Your life is at stake.

How can you ensure that you're one of the few who gets the best treatment?

Multiple reviews have shown that people who are seen by a gout specialist, typically a rheumatologist, get better treatment (in fact, they are 69% more likely to be taking the correct medication) and have fewer gout attacks and complications than those who are looked after just by their family doctor. They also have fewer trips to accident and emergency / ER. Despite this, less than 5% of people with gout attacks see a rheumatologist, and less than 60% of people with advanced gout and complications do so. If you aren't seeing a gout specialist, ask to be referred to one.

An American College of Rheumatologists expert panel concluded that patient education was key to people with gout getting their uric acid levels below 6 mg/dL (0.36 mmol/L) (and hence fewer gout attacks, and less chance of tophi, kidney stones and all the other complications). The person who understands the disease and how it should be treated is the person who gets the best treatment. That's why we wrote this book, and why you bought it.

In summary

What's the problem?	What should I do?
Doctors are overworked and can't know everything about every disease they are expected to treat. Only 1 in 10 people gets appropriately diagnosed. Perhaps half the people being treated for gout don't have it. Most people with gout don't get the proper treatment. Only a third of people get medication to lower their body's urate level, leaving the remaining two thirds at risk of tophi, kidney stones and joint damage. Of those who are treated, only about a quarter achieve target uric acid levels. At least two thirds of people don't take their medication correctly. Blood tests to check for serious drug complications are often not done. People on sub-optimal gout treatment have more gout attacks, more complications, and a 24% higher risk of dying - from any cause.	An American College of Rheumatologists expert panel concluded that the key to people getting the best treatment for their gout was patient education. You need to understand enough about the objectives and methods of gout treatment to take an active part in decisions about your care. You should be under the care of a rheumatologist or other doctor who specialises in gout. You should take all prescribed medicines correctly. Make sure you understand how what you eat and drink affects your urate level, and then keep to an appropriate diet. Keep a record of your attacks, medications and blood results so that you can spot trends and ensure tests are done on time.

Chapter 13

What do I need to know about the medicines used to treat gout?

In this chapter, you will find helpful information on the drugs commonly used in gout treatment. Decisions about which medication to use can be hugely complex. For example, the prescribing information for the non-steroidal anti-inflammatory drug indomethacin runs to 32 pages in the Physician's Desk Reference, the standard drug reference manual for US doctors. So, the information given here is no substitute for your doctor's careful evaluation of your particular circumstances – your age, what other medical conditions you have, what other medication you are taking, past adverse reactions to other drugs, etc. It does, however, act as a starting point for conversations with your doctor about your treatment choices.

Allopurinol

Use in gout: Allopurinol is used to lower the amount of urate in the body in order to reduce the risk of acute gout attacks and to get rid of tophi.

How allopurinol works: Allopurinol blocks the enzyme xanthine oxidase, which produces uric acid. Normal blood uric acid levels are usually achieved in one to three weeks. If allopurinol is stopped, blood uric acid returns to pre-treatment levels in 7 to 10 days

Dose: Allopurinol tablets are started at a dose of 100 mg once a day. The dose is increased at intervals of not less than one week, guided by the blood uric acid level. Most people take 200 mg or 300 mg once daily. Up to 400 mg to 600 mg may be needed, particularly in severe gout with tophi. Doses of 400 mg or more are given in divided doses rather than once a day.

The maximum daily dose is 800 mg.

What happens to allopurinol in the body: The effects of a dose of allopurinol last about 24 hours (hence you only need to take it once a day). It is excreted from the body in the urine.

Who should not take allopurinol: Anyone who has had a rash or other allergic reaction before when taking allopurinol should not take it again due to the risk of a severe reaction. In certain populations with a high risk of this allergic reaction, doctors will screen for a genetic marker of this risk (HLA-B*5801) before prescribing allopurinol. This genetic marker is most common in people with a Han Chinese, Korean or Thai background.

Precautions: Occasionally, allopurinol can cause liver inflammation, so blood tests to measure liver function are recommended for the first few months in patients with liver disease.

Occasionally allopurinol can prolong blood clotting times in patients taking certain anticoagulants such as warfarin and dicumarol. Such patients should have their clotting times measured periodically.

People with kidney impairment: People with impaired kidney function who are taking thiazide diuretics (such as bendroflumethiazide, hydrochlorthiazide and indapamide) are at an increased risk of developing severe allergic reactions with allopurinol and so should be monitored carefully. People with severely impaired kidney function may require a lower dose of allopurinol, longer intervals between doses, or both.

Pregnancy and breast-feeding: Taking any drugs during pregnancy or breast-feeding requires careful balancing of the risks and benefits and careful consultation with your doctor. Allopurinol passes into breast milk.

Adverse effects: The most severe side effect of allopurinol is an allergic reaction. This reaction typically begins as a rash, and if allopurinol is continued, it may progress to a more severe and even life-threatening reaction. Therefore, allopurinol should be stopped, and your doctor consulted if you develop a rash whilst taking allopurinol.

Sometimes an acute gout attack occurs as allopurinol begins to lower urate levels. The gout attack should be treated as usual. Allopurinol should be continued. Preventative treatment with either colchicine or non-steroidal anti-inflammatory drugs should be given for the first two to six months of treatment with allopurinol to reduce the risk of such attacks.

A few people have experienced drowsiness when starting allopurinol, so take care when driving or operating machinery until you understand how allopurinol affects you.

Uncommonly allopurinol can cause nausea and vomiting.

Some rare side effects have been reported, including bone marrow depression, fever, headache, tiredness, tingling and numbness and altered taste. If you are concerned you may have side effects from any medication, you should talk to your doctor.

Drug interactions: Some drugs appear to increase the risk of severe allergic reactions to allopurinol, including amoxicillin, ampicillin, bendroflumethiazide and other thiazide diuretics, and ACE inhibitors used to treat high blood pressure (captopril, enalapril, lisinopril, and other 'prils'). Some drugs increase the risk of bone marrow suppression, including azathioprine, mercaptopurine and ACE inhibitors (see above). This is far from a complete list of drugs that can interact with allopurinol, so talk to your doctor about your other medications before starting allopurinol.

Anakinra

Use in gout: Anakinra is used to treat acute gout attacks in patients who cannot take other treatments or in whom those treatments have failed.

How anakinra works: Anakinra acts as an anti-inflammatory by blocking a key inflammatory receptor on cells, the IL-1 receptor.

Dose: Anakinra is given by injection, 100 mg once daily, typically for five days, to treat a gout attack.

What happens to anakinra in the body: Anakinra is absorbed from the injection site, reaching peak blood levels in three to seven hours. It is excreted through the kidneys.

Who should not take anakinra: Because anakinra suppresses the immune system, it should not be taken by people with an active infection. If latent tuberculosis infection or hepatitis may be present, this should be investigated before anakinra is started.

Anakinra should not be used in people with a low white cell count.

Some authorities recommend that anakinra not be given to people with cancer.

Precautions: Anakinra should be used with caution in people with asthma as they appear to be at risk of developing severe infections.

Side effects are more common and can be more severe in the elderly.

Anakinra should be used with caution in people susceptible to recurrent infections.

People with kidney impairment: Because anakinra is excreted through the kidney, people with severe kidney impairment may need a reduced dose.

Pregnancy and breast-feeding: Taking any drugs during pregnancy or breast-feeding requires careful balancing of the risks and benefits and careful consultation with your doctor. There is insufficient evidence to assess the safety of anakinra in pregnancy. It is not known if anakinra passes into breast milk.

Adverse effects: Common side effects include headache, infections, low white blood cell count and low platelet count. Less commonly, it may cause skin reactions and rarely inflammation of the liver.

You should contact your doctor immediately if you develop signs suggestive of low white cells or platelets: fever, sore throat, bruising or bleeding.

Drug interactions: Because anakinra suppresses the immune system, live vaccines should not be given to people taking anakinra. The response to other vaccines may be less effective in someone taking anakinra.

Anakinra should not be given with other so-called 'biological' medicines that cause immunosuppression, including abatacept, certolizumab, etanercept, filgotinib and golimumab.

Canakinumab

Use in gout: Canakinumab is used to treat acute gout attacks in patients who cannot take other treatments or in whom those treatments have failed.

How canakinumab works: Canakinumab acts as an anti-inflammatory by blocking a key inflammatory receptor on cells, the IL-1 receptor.

Dose: Canakinumab is given as a single 150 mg injection. Another dose can be given after eight to twelve weeks if there has been a good response to the first, and another gout attack occurs.

What happens to canakinumab in the body: Canakinumab reaches peak blood levels about seven days after injection and stays in the body for a long time: after 26 days, the blood level is about half the peak level.

Who should not take canakinumab: Because canakinumab suppresses the immune system, it should not be taken by people with an active infection, including HIV, hepatitis B and hepatitis C. If there may be a possibility of latent tuberculosis infection or hepatitis, this should be investigated before canakinumab is started.

People with a low white cell count should not receive canakinumab.

Precautions: Canakinumab should be used with caution in people susceptible to recurrent infections.

Canakinumab should be used with caution in people with pre-existing cancer, as it is not clear if it may allow the cancer to progress.

People with kidney impairment: There is insufficient evidence to suggest if lower doses might be needed in people with kidney impairment.

Pregnancy and breast-feeding: Taking any drugs during pregnancy or breast-feeding requires careful balancing of the risks and benefits and careful consultation with your doctor. There is insufficient evidence to assess the safety of canakinumab in pregnancy. It is not known if canakinumab passes into breast milk.

Adverse effects: Common side effects include upper abdominal pain, joint pains, dizziness, vertigo, weakness, low white count and increased susceptibility to infection.

Drug interactions: Because canakinumab suppresses the immune system, live vaccines should not be given to people taking canakinumab. The response to other vaccines may be less effective in someone taking canakinumab.

There is an increased risk of severe bone marrow suppression if canakinumab is given together with anti-cancer chemotherapy drugs.

Colchicine

Use in gout: Colchicine is used to treat acute gout attacks and prevent further attacks.

How colchicine works: Colchicine has anti-inflammatory properties that act through several inflammatory processes. The onset of action is within 12 hours, with peak anti-inflammatory effects seen between 24 and 48 hours.

Dose: Some countries have 0.5 mg tablets and some 0.6 mg. This is the reason for the alternative doses given here.

To treat an acute gout attack, 1 mg or 1.2 mg of colchicine should be taken, followed by 0.5 mg or 0.6 mg one hour later. This dose should not be repeated for at least three days.

Patients already on colchicine to prevent gout attacks should wait 12 hours before re-starting their preventative dose.

To prevent future gout attacks, the dose is 0.5 mg or 0.6 mg once or twice daily

To treat an acute pseudogout attack, 0.5 mg or 0.6 mg should be taken three or four times daily.

To prevent further pseudogout attacks, the dose is 0.5 mg or 0.6 mg twice daily.

The maximum daily dose is 1.8 mg to treat an acute gout attack and 1.2 mg a day for attack prevention.

Colchicine is dangerous at higher doses. Keep colchicine tablets away from children.

What happens to colchicine in the body: Colchicine is rapidly absorbed from the gut and broken down by the liver. The ability to break down colchicine in the liver depends on the activity of certain enzymes, the levels of which vary between individuals and can be markedly affected by other drugs and even particular food and drinks.

Who should not take colchicine: People who have both kidney and liver impairment should not take colchicine. Some drugs affect the breakdown of colchicine in the liver, potentially leading to dangerously high levels. Anyone taking these drugs should not take colchicine (or should have the dose reduced to 50% or even 25% of a standard dose). These drugs include but are not limited to: a number of HIV drugs and antifungals; the antibiotics clarithromycin, ciprofloxacin, erythromycin and telithromycin; fluvoxamine, cyclosporine, verapamil and diltiazem.

Precautions: Do not drink grapefruit juice while taking colchicine, as grapefruit juice inhibits the enzyme that breaks down colchicine in the liver, leading to dangerously high levels.

The dose of colchicine may need to be reduced in the elderly, who are more susceptible to its side effects.

The dose of colchicine may need to be reduced in patients with liver impairment or gall bladder obstruction.

Colchicine should be used with caution in people with bone marrow suppression, as colchicine may make this worse.

People with kidney impairment: The dose of colchicine should be reduced in people with significant kidney impairment. Colchicine is not removed by dialysis.

Pregnancy and breast-feeding: Taking any drugs during pregnancy or breast-feeding requires careful balancing of the risks and benefits and careful consultation with your doctor. Colchicine causes birth defects when given to pregnant animals. The risk may be less in humans, but pregnant women should only use colchicine if the benefit greatly outweighs the risk. Colchicine passes into breast milk.

Adverse effects: Common side effects include nausea and vomiting, abdominal pain and diarrhoea. Less common side-effects include bone marrow suppression, hair loss, liver and kidney toxicity, nerve and muscle disorders and low sperm count.

Drug interactions: The breakdown of colchicine by the liver can be inhibited by some drugs and this can lead to potentially toxic levels of colchicine in the body. Therefore, it is essential to talk to your doctor about all the medication you take, including herbal medicines and other supplements, before any decision is taken to prescribe colchicine or to add any new medicines while you are taking colchicine.

Febuxostat

Use in gout: Febuxostat is used as an alternative to allopurinol to reduce urate levels in the body to prevent future gout attacks and get rid of tophi. There is an increased risk of cardiovascular death in people with pre-existing cardiovascular disease who take febuxostat. Therefore, febuxostat is only used for people in whom allopurinol has not worked or who cannot take allopurinol.

How febuxostat works: Febuxostat blocks the enzyme xanthine oxidase, which produces uric acid. Blood uric acid levels fall for about seven days after starting treatment before settling to their new level.

Dose: Febuxostat is started at a dose of 40 mg once a day. If after two weeks the blood uric acid level is still more than 6 mg/dL / 0.36 mmol/l, the dose may be increased to 80 mg once daily.

The maximum dose is 80 mg once a day. In the U.K., doses of up to 120 mg are prescribed.

What happens to febuxostat in the body: About half of a dose of febuxostat is absorbed from the gut. Over 24 hours, about half is excreted in the urine and half in the faeces.

Who should not take febuxostat: If you take azathioprine or mercaptopurine, you should not take febuxostat.

You should not take febuxostat if your uric acid levels are well controlled with allopurinol.

Precautions: Studies have shown a higher risk of sudden cardiovascular death in patients taking febuxostat than those taking allopurinol. Therefore, febuxostat should only be taken by people who cannot take allopurinol.

Febuxostat should be used with caution in people with pre-existing cardiovascular disease or who have had a stroke because of the increased risk of sudden cardiovascular death.

People who have had severe allergic reactions to allopurinol are at increased risk of developing similar reactions to febuxostat.

Febuxostat should be used with caution in people with severe liver disease.

People with kidney impairment: The dose of febuxostat should be reduced for people with severe kidney impairment.

Pregnancy and breast-feeding: Taking any drugs during pregnancy or breast-feeding requires careful balancing of the risks and benefits and careful consultation with your doctor. There is insufficient evidence to assess the safety of febuxostat in pregnancy. Febuxostat passes into the breast milk of animals, but this has not been investigated in humans.

Adverse effects: People taking febuxostat are at an increased risk of sudden cardiovascular death compared to people taking allopurinol. This risk is higher in people who have cardiovascular disease or have had a stroke.

Some people develop a rash with febuxostat, and this can become serious. Febuxostat should be stopped if you develop a severe rash.

Sometimes an acute gout attack occurs as febuxostat begins to lower urate levels. The gout attack should be as usual. Febuxostat should be continued. Preventative treatment with either colchicine or non-steroidal anti-inflammatory drugs should be given for the first two to six months of taking febuxostat to reduce the risk of such attacks.

Common side effects include diarrhoea, nausea, headache, abnormal liver blood tests and skin reaction.

A wide range of uncommon or rare side effects has been reported.

Drug interactions: Febuxostat can increase the blood levels of azathioprine and mercaptopurine, so it should not be given with either of them. Febuxostat should be used cautiously with other anti-cancer drugs due to the risk of kidney damage or kidney stone formation during chemotherapy.

Lesinurad

Use in gout: Lesinurad is used to reduce the amount of urate in the body and thus reduce the risk of future attacks. It is only used in people who have not reached target uric acid levels with allopurinol or febuxostat alone. It must be taken in combination with allopurinol or febuxostat.

How lesinurad works: Lesinurad increases the amount of urate excreted by the kidneys.

Dose: Lesinurad is taken as a once-daily dose of 200mg. It must be given in combination with either allopurinol or febuxostat and taken at the same time.

If you forget to take a dose of lesinurad, don't take it later in the day. Wait until the next day and take your usual dose with your allopurinol or febuxostat.

What happens to lesinurad in the body: Lesinurad is quickly and completely absorbed from the gut. It is mainly excreted in the urine.

Who should not take lesinurad: You should not take lesinurad if your urate levels can be controlled with allopurinol or febuxostat alone. You should not take lesinurad if your allopurinol dose is less than 300 mg per day.

You should not take lesinurad if you have severe kidney disease.

Precautions: Kidney toxicity was seen in clinical studies, particularly when lesinurad was used alone. It is important to keep well hydrated when taking lesinurad – drink at least 2 litres / 3 ½ pints per day.

Lesinurad is not recommended for people with severe liver impairment.

People with kidney impairment: You should not take lesinurad if you have severe kidney impairment, but it may be used if you have mild to moderate kidney disease.

Pregnancy and breast-feeding: Taking any drugs during pregnancy or breast-feeding requires careful balancing of the risks and benefits and careful consultation with your doctor. There is insufficient evidence to assess the safety of lesinurad in pregnancy. There is no information about whether lesinurad passes into breast milk.

Adverse effects: Side effects of lesinurad include kidney toxicity. Blood tests should be done regularly to measure kidney function. If these results worsen, lesinurad should be stopped and the cause investigated.

An increase in the rate of heart attacks and strokes was seen in the clinical trials.

The most common side effects of lesinurad are headache, nasal congestion, flu-like symptoms and heartburn.

Sometimes an acute gout attack occurs as lesinurad begins to lower urate levels. The gout attack should be treated as usual. Lesinurad should be continued. Preventative treatment with colchicine, or a non-steroidal anti-inflammatory drug, may be given for the first two to six months of treatment with lesinurad to reduce the risk of such attacks.

Drug interactions: Lesinurad may reduce the effectiveness of hormonal contraceptives in women. You should use alternative / additional contraceptive measures when taking lesinurad.

Lesinurad decreases the blood levels of the blood pressure drug nisoldipine and the HIV drug velpatasvir and may make them ineffective. These two medicines should not be taken with lesinurad.

Lesinurad can affect the blood levels of many other medicines. Be sure to talk to your doctor about all the other medicines you take, or start whilst taking lesinurad.

Non-steroidal anti-inflammatory drugs (NSAIDs)

Use in gout: Non-steroidal anti-inflammatory drugs are used to treat acute gout attacks and prevent recurrent attacks.

How NSAIDs work: Non-steroidal anti-inflammatory drugs block the production of chemicals called prostaglandins involved in inflammation.

Dose: The dose depends on which of the many non-steroidal anti-inflammatory drugs you are taking. See Table 5 on page 32.

What happens to NSAIDs in the body: The individual characteristics vary since there are numerous NSAIDs. In general, NSAIDs are well absorbed from the stomach reaching peak blood concentrations in two to four hours. Most of a dose is excreted in the urine, so people with poorly functioning kidneys can accumulate toxic levels.

Who should not take NSAIDs: Anyone who has had recurrent gastro-intestinal bleeding should not take NSAIDs.

Anyone who has had an allergic reaction or asthma/wheezing when taking aspirin (or other salicylates) or NSAIDs should not take non-steroidal anti-inflammatory drugs.

Anyone who has had a previous severe skin reaction to NSAIDs should not take them again.

Anyone who has had a recent coronary artery bypass graft, heart attack or stroke should not take NSAIDs.

Anyone with severe heart failure should not take NSAIDs.

Precautions: People who have had a stomach or duodenal ulcer or previous gastro-intestinal bleeding are at a 10-fold increased risk of having further G.I. bleeding if they take non-steroidal anti-inflammatory drugs. This risk is increased further by alcohol, smoking, anticoagulants, steroids, certain antidepressants (the SSRIs) and being elderly.

Non-steroidal anti-inflammatory drugs increase the risk of heart attacks and strokes in people with and without prior coronary heart disease or strokes. Therefore, they should be used with caution in people with known coronary heart disease or stroke as they are already at increased risk.

Non-steroidal anti-inflammatory drugs should be used with caution in people with high blood pressure as they can raise it further.

You should not take more than one NSAID at a time as this will increase the risk of harmful side effects. Many over the counter medicines contain NSAIDs. If in doubt, ask a doctor or pharmacist.

People with kidney impairment: Non-steroidal anti-inflammatory drugs are not recommended for people with severe kidney impairment as they can cause worsening of kidney function.

Pregnancy and breast-feeding: Taking any drugs during pregnancy or breast-feeding requires careful balancing of the risks and benefits and careful consultation with your doctor. Non-steroidal anti-inflammatory drugs should not be given after the 30th week of pregnancy as they can interfere with the normal development of the lung blood supply in the foetus. NSAIDs pass into breast milk. If necessary, it may be possible to breast-feed whilst taking NSAID, but this needs to be discussed first with the doctor.

Adverse effects: NSAIDs commonly cause gastro-intestinal inflammation and may cause ulceration and bleeding (see Precautions).

NSAIDs increase the risk of heart attacks and strokes (see Precautions).

NSAIDs can worsen heart failure and raise blood pressure.

NSAIDs may interfere with the release of eggs from the ovary leading to reversible fertility difficulties.

Other reported side effects include asthma/wheezing, indigestion, nausea, vomiting, constipation, diarrhoea, drowsiness and fatigue, dizziness, tinnitus, headache, depression, disturbed sleep, muscle pains and weakness, tingling and numbness, fluid retention, kidney impairment and bone marrow suppression.

Drug interactions: You should not take more than one NSAID at a time as this will increase the risk of harmful side effects. Many over the counter medicines contain NSAIDs. If in doubt, ask a doctor or pharmacist.

NSAIDs and steroids (prednisolone etc.) should generally not be taken together as this increases the likelihood of gastro-intestinal inflammation and bleeding.

NSAIDs and certain types of antidepressants (SSRIs such as citalopram, fluoxetine, fluvoxamine, paroxetine, duloxetine and venlafaxine) should generally not be taken together as this increases the likelihood of gastro-intestinal inflammation and bleeding.

When NSAIDs are taken with certain antihypertensive drugs (ACE inhibitors and ACE receptor blockers such as captopril, enalapril, fosinopril, lisinopril, ramipril, quinapril, azilsartan, candesartan, losartan and valsartan, or beta-blockers such as atenolol, labetalol, metoprolol and propranolol), they may lead to a fall in blood pressure and also kidney damage. The risk is higher in the elderly and people who are dehydrated.

Probenecid can block the excretion of NSAIDs by the kidney leading to potentially toxic blood levels. The dose of NSAIDs may need to be reduced.

Pegloticase

Use in gout: Pegloticase is used to lower urate levels in people with gout in whom other treatments have not been successful.

How pegloticase works: Pegloticase is a synthetic version of the enzyme uricase, which breaks down uric acid to the harmless, water-soluble chemical allantoin (often found in moisturisers). Most mammals have uricase, but it is missing in some higher primates, including humans.

Dose: Pegloticase is given by two-hour infusion at a dose of 8 mg every two weeks. An antihistamine, steroid and sometimes paracetamol/acetaminophen are given first to reduce the risk of allergic reactions.

What happens to pegloticase in the body: Pegloticase stays in the body for a long time after infusion, falling to half the peak blood level after two weeks.

Who should not take pegloticase: People who have had a previous allergic reaction to pegloticase and people with the G-6-PD enzyme deficiency should not receive pegloticase.

Precautions: Because of the risk of severe, even life-threatening allergic reactions, pegloticase should only be given at a specialised centre experienced in its use. The risk of such a reaction may be increased in people who re-start pegloticase treatment after a gap of four weeks or longer.

Uric acid levels should be closely measured during treatment. Levels above 6 mg/dL / 0.36 mmol/l may indicate treatment failure. In this case, pegloticase treatment should probably be stopped as patients with treatment failure are at a higher risk of allergic reactions.

People with a particular enzyme deficiency (G-6-PD deficiency) are at risk of severe anaemia if given pegloticase. Those at higher risk of this deficiency (including those with African, Mediterranean, Middle Eastern and South Asian ancestry) should be screened before starting pegloticase.

People with heart failure may develop a worsening of their condition with pegloticase.

People with kidney impairment: No dose reduction appears to be necessary for people with kidney impairment.

Pregnancy and breast-feeding: Taking any drugs during pregnancy or breast-feeding requires careful balancing of the risks and benefits and careful consultation with your doctor. There is insufficient evidence to assess the safety of pegloticase in pregnancy. It is not known if pegloticase passes into breast milk.

Adverse effects: The most concerning side effect of pegloticase is the risk of severe allergic reactions, as described above. Although the reactions most commonly occur around the time of the infusion, they may be delayed.

Sometimes an acute gout attack occurs as pegloticase begins to lower urate levels. The gout attack should be treated as usual. Pegloticase should be continued.

Drug interactions: Significant drug interactions have not been reported; however, urate-lowering drugs such as allopurinol, sulfinpyrazone and febuxostat are not given at the same time as pegloticase as they may mask a rise in uric acid levels that indicates pegloticase treatment failure. Any rise in uric acid levels must be detected early as those with pegloticase treatment failure are at increased risk of allergic reactions.

Prednisolone/prednisone (steroids)

Use in gout: Prednisolone or prednisone are used to treat an acute gout attack.

How steroids work: Steroids have anti-inflammatory effects through several mechanisms.

Dose: The most commonly used steroid tablets are prednisolone or prednisone. The usual dose for an acute gout attack is 20 mg to 30 mg either as a single dose or divided into two doses until the attack begins to resolve. The dose is then slowly reduced to zero over 7 to 10 days. The tablets should be taken with food to minimise stomach irritation.

What happens to steroids in the body: Peak blood levels occur after one to two hours. Prednisolone and prednisone are broken down by the liver and excreted by the kidneys. The effects of a single dose last two days or longer.

Who should not take steroids: The decision to prescribe steroids is a balance of risks and benefits.

Precautions: Anyone who may have latent tuberculosis should be screened before starting long courses of steroids. Steroids may suppress the immune response to many infections.

Steroids should be used with caution in people with:

- Heart failure, or who have had a recent heart attack.
- Active stomach or duodenal ulcers.
- Psychosis or emotional instability.
- Seizures/epilepsy.
- Diabetes, as they may increase blood sugar.
- Myasthenia gravis.
- Strokes or DVTs.

People with kidney impairment: People with kidney impairment can usually take a standard dose of prednisolone or prednisone.

Pregnancy and breast-feeding: Taking any drugs during pregnancy or breast-feeding requires careful balancing of the risks and benefits and careful consultation with your doctor. Because steroids are so widely prescribed, there is some information on the safety of steroids in pregnancy. The risks are considered relatively low, but long term treatment can cause growth retardation of the foetus. Steroids do cross into breast milk and can suppress growth. When steroids are essential, this risk can be managed by the timing of breast-feeding.

Adverse effects: Common side effects include anxiety, mood alteration, behavioural changes, sleep disturbance, confusion, tiredness, fluid retention, indigestion, nausea, and weight gain. Less commonly, steroids, particularly longer courses, can cause suppression of the body's normal steroid production, bone fractures, pancreatitis, cataracts and heart failure.

Drug interactions: Live vaccines should be used with caution in people receiving steroids.

Steroids and non-steroidal anti-inflammatory drugs should not be given together for prolonged periods because of the increased risk of gastric irritation.

Steroids may alter the effectiveness of:

- Anticoagulants such as warfarin.
- Oral contraceptives.
- Epilepsy medications such as carbamazepine and phenytoin
- Drugs for diabetes

There is a very long list of drugs with which steroids can potentially interfere. For this reason, you must tell your doctor about all the medicines you take, including herbal preparations and supplements, before starting prednisolone or prednisone.

Probenecid

Use in gout: Probenecid is used to reduce the amount of urate in the body and thus reduce the risk of future attacks.

How probenecid works: Probenecid increases the amount of urate excreted by the kidneys.

Dose: Probenecid is started at a dose of 250 mg twice a day, then increased to 500 mg twice a day after a week. If necessary, the dose can be increased by 500 mg daily every month to a maximum of 500 mg four times a day.

What happens to probenecid in the body: Probenecid is well absorbed from the gut and is excreted by the kidneys.

Who should not take probenecid: People with a previous allergic reaction to probenecid should not take it again.

People with uric acid kidney stones should not take probenecid since it increases the amount of uric acid in the urine, making the situation worse.

People with haematological (blood) problems should generally not take probenecid as there is a risk they could get worse.

Precautions: People with stomach or duodenal ulcers should take probenecid with caution as it may worsen their ulcers.

You should drink plenty of fluids while taking probenecid to reduce the risk of kidney stones.

People with kidney impairment: People with moderate or severe kidney impairment should generally not take probenecid.

Pregnancy and breast-feeding: Taking any drugs during pregnancy or breast-feeding requires careful balancing of the risks and benefits and careful consultation with your doctor. There is insufficient evidence to assess the safety of probenecid in pregnancy. Probenecid passes into breast milk at low concentrations.

Adverse effects: Side effects of probenecid include headache, upset stomach, vomiting, loss of appetite, dizziness, skin rashes, bone marrow suppression and severe allergic reactions.

Sometimes an acute gout attack occurs as probenecid begins to lower urate levels. The gout attack should be treated as usual. Probenecid should be continued. Preventative treatment with colchicine, but not non-steroidal anti-inflammatory drugs, may be given for the first two to six months of treatment with probenecid to reduce the risk of such attacks.

Drug interactions: Because of the effects probenecid has on the kidney, it can reduce the excretion of many other drugs, potentially causing toxicity. Before starting probenecid, you must tell your doctor about all your medicines, including herbal preparations and supplements. You must also tell your doctor that you take probenecid before starting any other medication.

While taking probenecid, do not take aspirin (or other salicylates, including Pepto-Bismol, Kaopectate and Maalox Total Relief).

Probenecid reduces the excretion of non-steroidal anti-inflammatory drugs, so these are best avoided while taking probenecid.

Sulfinpyrazone/sulphinpyrazone

Use in gout: Sulfinpyrazone is used to reduce the amount of urate in the body and hence to reduce the risk of future attacks.

How sulfinpyrazone works: Sulfinpyrazone increases the amount of urate excreted by the kidneys.

Dose: Sulfinpyrazone is usually started at 100 mg or 200 mg once a day. The dose can be increased every few days up to 800 mg per day, guided by the change in uric acid levels.

What happens to sulfinpyrazone in the body: Sulfinpyrazone is rapidly absorbed from the gut and then excreted through the kidney.

Who should not take sulfinpyrazone: Sulfinpyrazone should not be taken by people with ongoing stomach or duodenal ulceration, significant gastric irritation, or haematological (blood) disorders.

Precautions: You should drink plenty of fluids while taking sulfinpyrazone to reduce the risk of kidney stones.

People with kidney impairment: Little information is available, but dose adjustments may be required for people with kidney impairment.

Pregnancy and breast-feeding: Taking any drugs during pregnancy or breast-feeding requires careful balancing of the risks and benefits and careful consultation with your doctor. There is insufficient evidence to assess the safety of sulfinpyrazone in pregnancy. It is not known if sulfinpyrazone passes into breast milk.

Adverse effects: Common side effects include lower back pain and painful urination, and sometimes a skin rash. Rare side effects include shortness of breath, mouth ulcers, bone marrow suppression, kidney stones, kidney toxicity and allergic reactions.

Sometimes an acute gout attack occurs as sulfinpyrazone begins to lower urate levels. The gout attack is treated as usual. Sulfinpyrazone should be continued. Preventative treatment with either colchicine or non-steroidal anti-inflammatory drugs should be given for the first two to six months of treatment with sulfinpyrazone to reduce the risk of such attacks.

Drug interactions: Because of the effects sulfinpyrazone has on the kidney, it can reduce the excretion of lots of other drugs, potentially causing toxicity. You must tell your doctor about all the medicines you take, including herbal preparations and supplements, before starting sulfinpyrazone. You must also tell your doctor that you are taking sulfinpyrazone before starting any other medication.

While taking sulfinpyrazone, do not take aspirin (or other salicylates, including Pepto-Bismol, Kaopectate and Maalox Total Relief).

Sulfinpyrazone may affect the activity of anticoagulants such as warfarin.

Understanding your medication

Whenever you are prescribed a new medicine, it is vital that you understand why you have been prescribed it and how you should take it.

You can get this information from your doctor, a pharmacist and from the information leaflet that should come with your medicine.

You should know the answers to these questions:

- What is the name of the medicine?
- What is the dose?
- How many times a day should I take it?
- Do I need to take it with food or on an empty stomach?
- What should I do if I miss a dose?
- What should I do if I accidentally take too much?
- Are there any side effects?
- Is it okay to take this medication with my other medicines?
- For how long will I need to take this medicine?
- If the medicine is a painkiller, you should also ask, “What should I do if I’m taking the maximum dose and still in pain.”

Chapter 14

How will I know if I have kidney stones?

Because urate is excreted in the urine, and because it is poorly soluble and so can crystallise in the urine, around 20% (one in five) of people with gout develop kidney stones. Whether they are aware of it though depends on how big the stones are and where they are.

A kidney stone that is too large to pass into the ureter (the tube that goes from the kidney to the bladder) will remain in the kidney and typically causes no symptoms.

Tiny stones will pass easily down the ureter to the bladder and then will be passed in the urine. They may be noticed like little bits of gravel as you pass urine.

The worst kind of stones are the medium-sized ones, as these can get stuck in the ureter. As the muscles in the wall of the

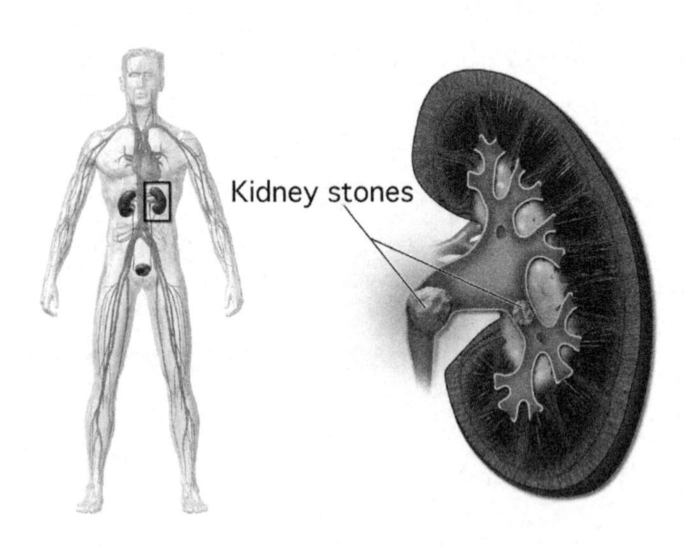

Figure 19: Kidney stones are common in gout.

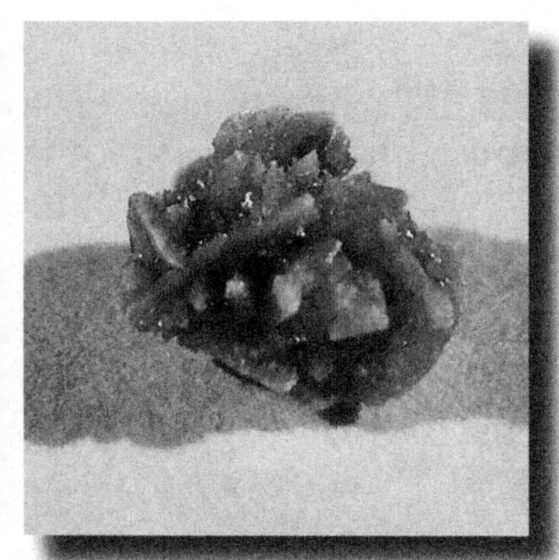

Figure 20: A uric acid kidney stone.

ureter contract to try to push the stone through, it causes exquisite pain. Where the pain is felt depends on where in the ureter the stone is stuck. It can be felt in the flank or kidney area radiating across the abdomen, down into the genital region, or just above the pubic bone. This pain is called renal colic and typically occurs intermittently, lasting between 20 minutes and an hour.

As you can see from the photograph, urate crystals are spiky. It's not hard to understand why they cause so much pain.

Characteristically, people with renal colic can't keep still. They tend to pace backwards and forward, sit down, stand up, and roll around – anything to relieve the pain. They may be ashen and are often sweating profusely. Nausea and vomiting are common.

Some people with renal colic pass urine frequently, sometimes just small amounts and the urine may be pink or even red with blood.

Kidney stones increase the risk of a urinary tract infection, with or without the pain of renal colic. Symptoms of a urinary tract infection include passing urine frequently, pain on passing urine, cloudy and sometimes smelly urine, and sometimes fever and chills.

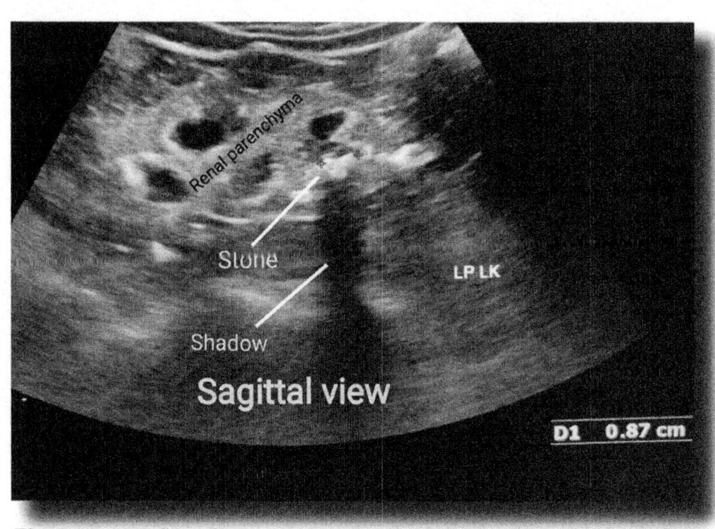

Figure 21: In this ultrasound scan, the kidney stone can be seen as a white spot just above centre. Because the ultrasound waves can't pass through it, it casts a shadow which can be clearly seen here.

Kidney stones may be seen on x-ray, CT scan, ultrasound, or a combination of these, depending on what they are made of. Pure urate stones can't be seen on x-ray (as they don't contain calcium), so although an abdominal x-ray is often done first, a normal x-ray can't rule out a stone.

A special kind of CT scan (a spiral or helical CT) is now thought to be the best way to see a kidney stone and also to see what effect it is having on the kidney, though not all hospitals have this type of CT scanner.

An ultrasound scan can also pick up a kidney stone and show the effects on the kidney. For example, the pressure of urine can build up behind a stone stuck in the ureter, which can distend the kidney.

Chapter 15

How are kidney stones treated?

Kidney stones that are composed solely of urate and which are not causing any problems may simply dissolve with good hydration (3 litres/6 pints a day) and medication to block the production of urate. (Drugs that increase urate excretion should be avoided as they increase the amount of urate in the urine and this can form new stones.) Sometimes the doctor may decide to help this process along by making the urine more alkaline so that the urate dissolves more quickly. This can be done with potassium citrate, acetazolamide or certain foods (See page 81).

For a stone that has become stuck in the ureter, the priority is pain control. Strong painkillers are required and are usually given first by injection for rapid results. If a urinary tract infection is present, that is also treated with antibiotics. Most people will eventually pass their kidney stones, often with the help of drugs like tamsulosin, terazosin or doxazosin, which relax the muscles of the ureter, allowing the stones to pass through.

If the stone does not pass out on its own, various methods can be used to get it out. The most commonly used procedure is shockwave lithotripsy, where high-intensity ultrasound waves are used to break up the stone so that it can be passed. Lithotripsy is successful in 80 to 85% of cases. Stones can also be removed using an endoscope (fibre-optic camera and instruments) passed into the urinary tract, usually through the bladder.

To prevent a recurrence, it is important to stay well hydrated and avoid purine-rich foods.

Chapter 16

How should my progress be monitored?

Acute attack

In an acute attack of gout, the most important considerations are controlling the pain and making sure there's nothing else going on.

If pain control is not adequate, then either an increase in dose or a change in medication should be considered.

Gout attacks usually settle in a few days. If an attack fails to resolve or feels significantly different from previous episodes, then further investigations may be necessary to make sure that the symptoms really are due to gout and only gout.

Reducing the frequency of attacks

After the first attack of gout, it is important to note how often further attacks occur. There may be no more or very few with a long time in between attacks. If attacks happen more than once a year, your doctor may decide to put you on daily preventative treatment with colchicine or a non-steroidal anti-inflammatory drug.

Your doctor will decide if you need medicines to lower the urate level in your body. The decision will be based on the frequency of attacks, your blood uric acid level, the presence of tophi or kidney stones, and your other medical conditions.

Keeping track of the attacks of gout, how long each episode lasts, and how their frequency changes with treatment is vital for making good decisions. You can use the charts at the back of this Handbook to record this information (page 198 and page 232).

Reducing the amount of urate in the body

If a decision is made to reduce the amount of urate in the body, it is important to monitor the urate load by measuring the blood uric acid level. It should be measured before any treatment is started. Treatment with a urate-lowering drug is started at a low dose to avoid bringing on an attack. Uric acid levels are then measured, and the dose of the medicine is increased step by step until the target uric acid levels are reached. This may mean monthly blood tests for uric acid until the correct dose has been determined.

Reaching the appropriate target level of uric acid in the blood is vital to reducing the risk of attacks and long-term complications. The recommended target levels are 0.6 mg/dL (0.36 mmol/L) for someone without tophi, and 0.5 mg/dL (0.30 mmol/L) for someone with tophi. Around 80% of people with gout never reach their target level. You need to work with your doctor (badger them if necessary – don't be shy) to ensure that your uric acid levels are measured regularly and that changes are made to your medication until you reach these target levels.

Once a stable, effective dose of allopurinol or another urate-lowering medicine has been achieved, the blood uric acid level is usually measured at least once a year to ensure the medication continues to be effective. Every six months is probably better. You can use the charts at the back of this Handbook to record this information (page 214 and page 232).

Getting rid of tophi

Tophi usually shrink and disappear once the amount of urate in the body has been reduced. In order to monitor this process, you can use the tables and charts at the back of the Handbook to record the details of any tophi you may have (page 218 and page 232).

Monitoring the kidneys

Since gout can cause kidney stones, and kidney stones can sometimes cause kidney damage, it is advisable to check kidney function every so often. This is done primarily by measuring urea/blood urea nitrogen (BUN) and creatinine levels in the blood. It is particularly important for people who already have kidney disease and for those taking non-steroidal anti-inflammatory drugs (NSAIDs) and certain other medicines, as these can impair kidney function too.

How often kidney function should be measured depends on many factors, including whether you have kidney stones, your age, other medical conditions, and what medications you are taking. Ideally, it should be measured at least once a year but may need to be done more often. You can record the results of these blood tests in the tables and charts at the back of this Handbook (page 232).

Monitoring the side-effects of medication

Certain drugs given for gout can cause side-effects that may be picked up early and effectively through blood tests. How often these tests should be done depends very much on your individual circumstances, other medical conditions you may have, and any other medicines you may be taking. Table 9 lists the normally recommended tests for medicines taken for gout.

	Kidney tests	Liver tests	Blood count
Allopurinol	✓	✓	✓
Anakinra	✓		✓
Canakinumab			✓
Colchicine	✓	✓	✓
Febuxostat	✓	✓	
Lesinurad	✓		
NSAIDs	✓		✓
Pegloticase			
Prednisolone			
Probenecid	✓		
Sulphinpyrazone	✓		

Table 9: Recommended blood tests for gout medicines – frequency and timing of tests depends on many things. Talk to your doctor to find out how often you should have these tests.

Chapter 17

How will I know if my medication needs changing?

During the treatment of a gout attack, it is easy to tell if the medication is working or not. At this stage, treatment is about getting the pain under control while the episode resolves over a few days. If the pain is not well controlled, you should first try physical measures such as resting the joint, ice packs and splinting. If these do not help, you should talk to your doctor about the best next step. If you are being treated with NSAIDs, this could mean adding paracetamol/acetaminophen or increasing the dose of NSAIDs. If you are being treated with colchicine, it may be possible to increase the colchicine dose, or an NSAID may be added.

In order to avoid long-term complications, it is common to reduce the amount of urate in the body, and monitor progress by checking blood uric acid levels, so that the dose of preventative drugs can be optimised. Unfortunately, many people are undertreated because they are just prescribed a standard dose, particularly with allopurinol. Preventive treatment is guided by regular blood uric acid tests (monthly initially, then six-monthly or annually once the dose has been stabilised), monitoring the frequency of attacks, and the presence and size of tophi

You should talk to your doctor about increasing the dose of preventative medicine or changing to a different one if the frequency of attacks has not reduced, if tophi are not getting smaller after six months of treatment, or if your blood uric acid level is not in the target range. Generally speaking, the lower the level, the better. Table 10 shows the target blood uric acid levels.

Target uric acid level	
No tophi	< 6 mg/dL (0.36 mmol/L)
Tophi present	< 5 mg/dL (0.30 mmol/L)

Table 10: Target uric acid levels on preventative treatment

Significant drug side effects are also a reason to change medication. Important side-effects of drugs are discussed in the section What Do I Need to Know About the Medicines Used to Treat Gout (Chapter 13 on page 49) and are summarised in Table 11.

Medication	Side effects that may require a change in treatment
Allopurinol	▲ Rash, fever and/or jaundice (yellowing of the skin and eyes) ▲ Bone marrow suppression – suggested by fever, sore throat, bruising or bleeding Abnormal liver function tests
Anakinra	▲ Bone marrow suppression – suggested by fever, sore throat, bruising or bleeding
Canakinumab	▲ Bone marrow suppression – suggested by fever, sore throat, bruising or bleeding
Colchicine	▲ Bone marrow suppression – suggested by fever, sore throat, bruising or bleeding ▲ Jaundice (yellowing of the skin and eyes) Abnormal kidney function tests Abnormal liver function tests
Febuxostat	▲ Jaundice (yellowing of the skin and eyes) ▲ Chest pain or heart attack Abnormal liver function tests
Lesinurad	Abnormal kidney function tests

Medication	Side effects that may require a change in treatment
Non-steroidal anti-inflammatory drugs	▲ Severe indigestion, vomiting blood or 'coffee grounds', black stools ▲ Chest pain or heart attack Abnormal kidney function tests
Pegloticase	▲ Allergic reactions Worsening heart failure
Steroids	Making diabetes difficult to control
Probenecid	▲ Bone marrow suppression – suggested by fever, sore throat, bruising or bleeding
Sulphinpyrazone	Abnormal kidney function tests
	▲: Consult your doctor immediately

Table 11: Red flags to talk to your doctor about changing medication due to side effects.

Chapter 18

What questions should I ask the doctor at follow-up visits?

This book aims to provide you with information and understanding so that you can talk with confidence to your doctor and understand the decisions they make. The questions suggested here are meant as openings for discussion so that you can understand and be involved in the decisions made about your health. To participate in those discussions, you should have read the appropriate sections in the Handbook.

Once a diagnosis of gout has been firmly established, and the acute attack has settled, the priorities are to reduce the number and frequency of future attacks and prevent or treat the complications of gout, namely tophi, kidney stones, and joint damage.

The frequency of attacks can be reduced by taking a lower dose of non-steroidal anti-inflammatory drugs (NSAIDs) or colchicine every day, and often, but not always, a drug like allopurinol to reduce the amount of urate in the body. You might ask your doctor, "**What do you recommend to reduce the risk and frequency of future attacks.**" (see page 34).

You should also ask, "**What should I do if I feel another attack coming on?**" Ideally, your doctor will prescribe you a course of treatment to begin as soon as you feel an attack starting. The treatment of a gout attack is much more effective if it is started early.

Even if you only have attacks rarely, it is possible that urate crystals are being deposited in your joints, kidneys and other tissues, storing up problems for the future. To see if you are at risk of this, you should have your blood uric acid levels measured. If your doctor has not done this within a month or two of your first attack, you should ask, "**Would it be**

possible to have my blood uric acid level measured to see if I need treatment to reduce it?"

Suppose attacks continue to occur frequently and you have not been put on medication to reduce the amount of urate in the body. In that case, it will be appropriate to ask, **"Do you think now is the time to start some medication to reduce my urate level?"**

Once you are on medication to reduce the amount of urate in the body and hence dissolve tophi or kidney stones, it is essential to measure the amount of uric acid in the blood regularly in order to get the dose right. Usually, this is done before starting treatment, then once a month or so until the most effective dose has been found, and then once or twice a year to make sure it continues working. You could ask the doctor, "How will you find the most effective dose for me" and, **"How often will you measure my blood uric acid level while I'm on treatment?"**

The next time you see the doctor after having a blood or urine test for uric acid, you should ask them for the result. There is space at the back of this Handbook to record the results. If your blood uric acid level is not in the target range (0.6 mg/dL (0.36 mmol/L) if you don't have tophi, 0.5 mg/dL (0.30 mmol/L) if you do), you should ask your doctor, **"What are we going to do to get my uric acid level down to the target range?"**

If you have tophi, once you are put on medication to reduce the amount of urate in the body, you should see the tofi getting smaller within six months or so. If you don't see them shrinking, you should ask, **"My tophi don't seem to be getting smaller, and it's been .... months since I started treatment to reduce the amount of urate in my body. Are you sure that these are tophi, and if so, do we need to change my medication?"**

If you have had kidney stones, you will probably have been seen by a kidney/urology specialist. It is worth asking, **"Do you know if I have any other stones in my kidneys, and if so, should we be doing something about them?"** (see page 68).

Many people with gout have other diseases such as cardiovascular disease, diabetes and high blood pressure. They may not be aware they have these conditions, so it is important to take the opportunity to be assessed for any other problems that may need attention. You can ask your doctor, **"I have heard that many people with gout have other medical conditions like high blood pressure, cardiovascular disease and diabetes. Would you mind giving me a check-up to ensure I don't have something I'm unaware of?"**

Chapter 19

What can I do for myself?

In addition to taking the medication prescribed by your doctor, there is plenty you can do for yourself to relieve the symptoms of a gout attack, reduce the risk of further attacks, and prevent complications such as joint damage and kidney stones.

Treatment of an acute attack

In addition to taking medication to treat gout, you should rest the affected joint(s). If movement of the joint is excruciating, you may get relief by splinting the joints to prevent movement. Ice packs can also provide pain relief when applied to the joints.

The easiest way to splint a big toe is to put some cotton wool between it and the second toe and then tape them together. Alternately, toe splints can be purchased.

A wrist is best splinted with a proper wrist splint, but you can improvise with folded newspaper or folded cardboard placed beneath the wrist and then held in place with strips of cloth tied around the board and arm.

Elbows and shoulders can be rested by placing the arm in a sling.

For other joints, a commercial splint or brace made for that specific joint is the easiest and most effective method of immobilizing the joint. If improvising temporarily, be careful that the splint is not tied on too tightly (to prevent impairment of circulation), and also ensure that the splint does not rub on the skin and cause abrasions.

Prevention of future attacks and kidney stones:

Gout occurs because urate is not very soluble in blood and body fluids and so can crystallize in the tissues. Increasing the volume of water passing through your system can help dissolve more urate and remove it from the body via the urine. You should try to drink three litres/six pints of fluids daily. It doesn't have to be water; it could be any liquid food or drink (except beer!). However, urate is excreted much less efficiently if the urine is acidic, so you should mostly avoid food and beverages that acidify the urine. These include meat, fish and shellfish, eggs, fizzy drinks and alcohol. Conversely, food and drinks that alkalinize the urine will result in more urate being excreted. Try to include more of these in your diet.

Foods that alkalinise the urine Good for gout	
	Most fruits: apples, apricots, avocados, bananas, berries, dates, oranges, grapefruits, lemons, melon, cherries, figs, grapes, kiwi, mangoes, nectarines, peaches, pears, pineapples, raisins, rhubarb, tangerines – and their juices
	Most vegetables: asparagus, aubergine/eggplant, beets, broccoli, Brussels sprouts, cabbage, carrot, cauliflower, celery, chard, cauliflower, collard greens, cucumbers, green beans, kale, lettuce, mustard greens, onions, parsnips, peas, peppers, pumpkin, spinach, sweet potatoes, tomatoes, turnips and watercress
	Nuts and seeds: almonds, chestnuts, flax seeds, pumpkin seeds and sunflower seeds
	Dairy products: milk, cheese, cream and yoghurt
	Tofu and tempeh
	Whey protein powder

Table 12: Foods that alkalinise the urine and increase the excretion of urate.

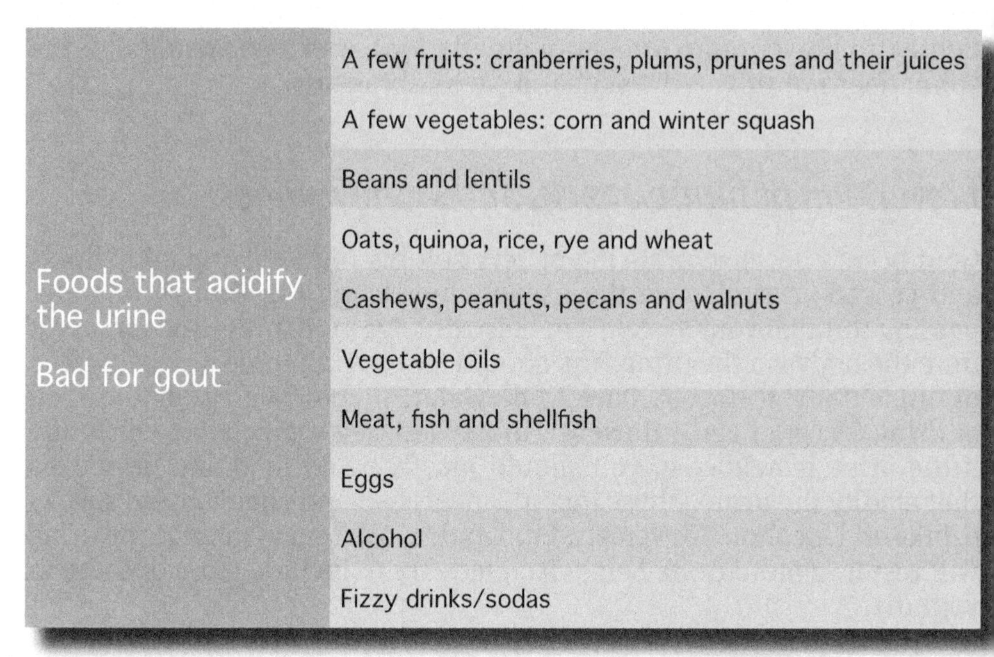

Foods that acidify the urine Bad for gout	A few fruits: cranberries, plums, prunes and their juices
	A few vegetables: corn and winter squash
	Beans and lentils
	Oats, quinoa, rice, rye and wheat
	Cashews, peanuts, pecans and walnuts
	Vegetable oils
	Meat, fish and shellfish
	Eggs
	Alcohol
	Fizzy drinks/sodas

Table 13: Foods that acidify the urine and decrease the excretion of urate.

Urate is produced in the body by the breakdown of chemicals called purines, which are used to make DNA and RNA and other molecules used by the body to store and transport energy. Some of these purines come from within our own bodies, and some come from our diet. Figure 22 shows that the risk of recurrent gout attacks is related to daily purine intake. The risk of gout attacks rises sharply once the daily purine intake exceeds about 1000 mg (1 gram). Therefore, it makes sense to reduce the amount of purine-rich foods eaten. Restricting purine-rich foods in the diet can lower blood uric acid levels by about 1 mg/dL (0.06 mmol/litre).

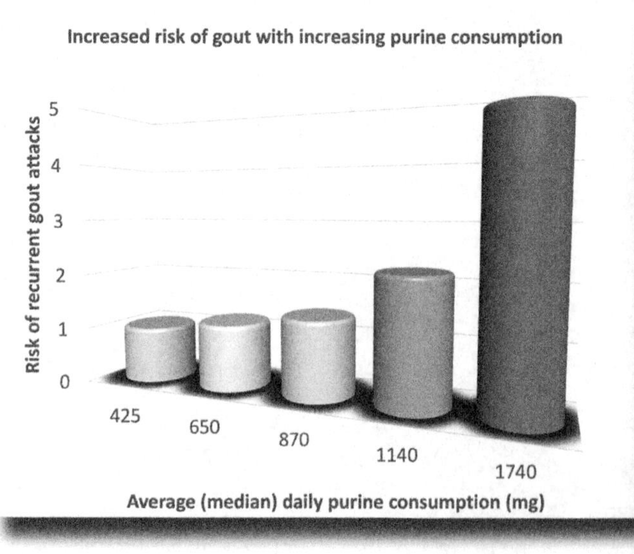

Figure 22: Eating lots of purines greatly increases the risk of future gout attacks.

Table 14 overleaf shows the purine content of some representative foods. The numbers refer to the purine content in milligrams per 100g of each foodstuff. Foods that are low in purines are foods that are generally considered healthy. Having a diet rich in these foods will also help you maintain a healthy weight and reduce the risk of many other diseases, including heart attacks, stroke and cancer. To reduce the frequency of gout attacks, you should try to get most of your protein from plant sources. Some authorities recommend that people with gout keep their daily purine intake below 400 mg. As Figure 22 demonstrates, a daily intake of 1000 mg or more dramatically increases the likelihood of having further gout attacks. People with the highest level of purine consumption have five times higher risk of gout further attacks. Lots of gout-specific recipe books are available on Amazon and elsewhere.

When using this table to make food choices, remember to consider the amount you eat. The numbers refer to the amount of purine in milligrams in 100g (3.5 oz) of each food. You're likely to drink a lot of beer, but it takes a particular person to eat 100g of dried anchovies.

High fructose corn syrup, used as a sweetener in many foods and drinks, should be avoided. Eating or drinking 70 g of high fructose corn syrup (the amount contained in a little less than two cans of cola or similar) will raise the blood level of uric acid in an average-sized man by 1 to 2 mg/dL (0.06 to 0.12 mmol/L) within two hours. In one study from New Zealand, people who drank four servings of sugar-sweetened soft drinks each day had an almost seven times higher risk of gout than those who consumed none.

Vitamin C supplements are often recommended to prevent attacks of gout. There is an association between higher levels of vitamin C in the blood and lower urate levels. However, a recent, comprehensive review of the subject concluded that there is insufficient data from well-conducted studies to recommend taking vitamin C supplements. Better advice would be to eat a diet rich in fruit and vegetables, which not only provides vitamin C but also reduces the risk of further gout attacks in multiple ways, helps maintain a healthy weight, and offers multiple other health benefits.

Gout is more common in people who are overweight and even more so in people whose obesity has caused a derangement of the body's metabolism, called metabolic syndrome. In one study, losing just 5 kg (11 lb) reduced blood uric acid by 1.1 mg/dL / 0.07 mmol/L. So, if you are overweight, now is the perfect time to look at your eating and exercise routines and make the changes needed to start losing weight and keeping it off.

Eggs	0	Walnuts	17	Spinach - old leaf	51
Milk	0	Red cabbage	17	Leg of lamb	51
Mayonnaise	0	Leeks	17	Soy sauce	55
Tea and coffee	0	Garlic	17	Chickpeas/Garbanzo	56
Wine	0	Sweet potato	17	Cauliflower	57
Honey	1	White bread	18	Corned beef	57
Butter	1	Green beans	18	Haddock	59
Margarine	1	Avocado	18	Frankfurter sausage	61
Strawberry	2	Pasta	20	Bacon	62
Carrot	2	Shiitake - fresh	21	Peas	63
Onion	2	Soy milk	22	Veal meat	63
Banana	3	Herring roe	22	Minced beef	64
Cabbage	3	Sunflower seeds	25	Miso	64
Pumpkin	3	Brussel sprouts	25	Asparagus	65
Fruit jam	3	Chocolate	25	Deer meat	65
Tomatoes	4	Wheat flour	26	Duck meat	67
Salmon roe	4	Wholemeal bread	27	Green bell pepper	69
Alcohol-free beer	4	Potato chips/crisps	29	Broccoli	70
Yoghurt	5	Almonds	31	Monkfish	70
Lettuce	5	Tofu	31	Rabbit	71
Lager	5	Salted peanuts	33	Cod	71
Cheese	6	Ketchup	33	Ham	74
Apple	6	Cornflakes	34	Buckwheat flour	76
Wheat beer	6	Semolina	34	Beef sirloin	77
Fruit juices	7	Peach	34	Scallop	77
Potato	7	Broad beans	36	Beef brisket	79
Oranges	8	Bean sprouts	36	Pork shoulder	81
Cucumber	9	Rice	37	Pork loin	83
Plums	10	Oyster mushrooms	38	Lentils - cooked	84
Olives	10	Okra	40	Cow stomach	84
Malt beer/lager	10	Barley	44	Pheasant	88
Sweetcorn	12	Vienna sausage	45	Cow tongue	90
Chanterelle mushrm	13	Prunes	46	Turkey meat	91
Courgette/Zucchini	13	Soybeans	48	Caviar	95
Barbecue sauce	15	Peanuts	49	Mutton	96
Kidney beans	16	Apricots - dried	49	Beef tenderloin	98
Hazelnuts	17	Aubergine/Eggplant	51	King crab	99

Lobster	102	Octopus	137	Oyster	185
Tongue	104	Herring	140	Pig kidney	195
Beef shin	106	Salami	146	Cow liver	220
Sea bass	107	Salmon - fresh	146	Lentils - dried	222
Sardines	109	Clam	146	Blackeye peas - dried	230
Chicken wing	113	Lamb's liver	147	Sardines - fresh	279
Pork rump	113	Crab	152	Pig liver	285
Fermented soybeans	114	Tuna	157	Chicken liver	312
Tuna - canned	117	Mackerel	165	Anchovies - canned	321
Pig heart	119	Prosciutto	168	Herring - canned	378
Pork tenderloin	120	Squid	170	Shiitake - dried	380
Chicken leg	123	Pinto beans - dried	171	Sardines - canned	399
Chicken heart	125	Spinach - young leaf	172	Whitebait - dried	472
Lamb chops	126	Chicken breast	172	Bonito - dried	493
Halibut	133	Cow kidney	174	Dried shrimp	749
Salmon - canned	133	Shrimp	180	Spirulina	1077
Oyster sauce	134	Rainbow trout	181	Anchovy - dried	1109
Beef topside	135	Cow heart	185	Yeast	2996

0 - 50mg/100g	Very low. Eat freely.
51 - 100 mg/100g	Low. Eat freely.
101 - 200 mg/100g	Medium. Eat sparingly.
201 - 300 mg/100g	High. Avoid.
> 301 mg/100g	Very high. Avoid.

Table 14: Purine content of some representative foods in milligrams of purine per 100g foodstuff. Within each category, the foodstuffs are listed in order of increasing purine content.

As we have discussed before, alcohol is a risk factor both for developing gout and for having further attacks. The risk of gout rises steeply with alcohol consumption of more than nine units per week, equivalent to nine single measures of spirits, four and a half pints of beer, or six small glasses of wine. However, even below this level, drinking alcohol contributes to raised urate levels in the body, so keep alcohol to a minimum.

Chapter 20

Under what circumstances should I see my doctor immediately?

After the first one or two attacks of gout, you will likely recognise subsequent attacks without difficulty, and you will have been advised by your doctor on what medication to take for an attack. However, you should see your doctor if an attack feels very different to the ones you've had before or if it is not settling down within a few days. Just because you have gout doesn't mean you can't get inflamed joints from other causes, including bacterial joint infections.

If you develop severe kidney or loin pain, which may spread across the abdomen or down into the lower abdominal or genital region and may be associated with frequent urination and/or blood in the urine, you may have a kidney stone. You should contact your doctor or go to the hospital emergency department.

Febuxostat and NSAIDs have been associated with an increased risk of cardiovascular disease. If you develop chest pain or tightness, you should contact your doctor immediately or go to the hospital emergency department. You could be having a heart attack.

If you are taking allopurinol or febuxostat and you get a rash, you should contact your doctor immediately and ask if you should stop the allopurinol. Sometimes the rash can progress quickly to a much more severe reaction.

If you are taking non-steroidal anti-inflammatory drugs and develop severe indigestion, vomit blood or 'coffee grounds', or pass black stools, you should contact your doctor immediately or go to the hospital emergency department. You could be bleeding from stomach inflammation or an ulcer caused by the drugs.

A small number of people taking febuxostat, colchicine or allopurinol have developed serious liver inflammation (hepatitis). You should see your doctor if you develop jaundice: yellowing of the skin and whites of the eyes and passing dark urine.

A very rare side effect of allopurinol, anakinra, canakinumab, colchicine and probenecid is suppression of the bone marrow. Once this becomes severe, the symptoms are fever, sore throat, bruising and bleeding. You should see your doctor immediately if you develop these symptoms.

Symptom	May be due to
Kidney or loin pain spreading across the abdomen or down into the genitals, and/or blood in the urine	Kidney stones
Severe indigestion, vomiting blood or 'coffee-grounds' or passing black stools	Bleeding from stomach inflammation or ulcer
A rash while taking allopurinol or febuxostat	Beginning of a severe reaction
An attack that isn't settling down in a few days	A joint infection
An attack that feels quite different from previous attacks	A joint infection
Chest pain or tightness, sweating and shortness of breath	A heart attack
Yellowing of the skin and eyes and passing dark urine	Jaundice from liver inflammation
Fever, sore throat, bruising and bleeding	Bone marrow suppression

Table 15: Contact your doctor if you have any of these symptoms.

Chapter 21

What is the long-term outlook with gout?

In the early stages of gout, the attacks settle on their own within a few days, and the symptoms can be well controlled with medication.

Some people will only ever have one attack of gout, others may have the occasional attack, but in some, urate crystals continue to be deposited in joints, kidneys, and other tissues. For these people, if no treatment is given, the future is likely to include continuing joint pains, tophi, kidney stones and possibly kidney damage.

Large accumulations of urate crystals are called tophi. If they are close to the skin, they can be felt and seen as white or yellow nodules. These are most common in the fingers, hands, elbows, feet, Achilles tendons and earlobes. Tophi can also occur in joints where they can damage the joint surfaces leading to persistent pain, a restricted range of movement at the joint, and joint deformity.

Because urate can crystallise in the urine and kidneys, about one in five people with gout develop kidney stones. Small stones can be excruciating as they pass down the ureter to the bladder. Larger stones can cause damage to the kidneys and impair kidney function.

With appropriate treatment to reduce the body's urate level, and regular monitoring of the uric acid level to ensure it stays within the target range, together with good hydration and eating an appropriate diet, the risk of these long-term complications can be significantly reduced.

People who develop gout at an earlier age, that is before middle-age, often have a more aggressive form of gout. Their uric acid levels may be more difficult to control and joint damage is more likely.

Looking at the bigger picture, we know that people with gout are also likely to have other medical conditions. As we discussed earlier, many people with gout also have high blood pressure and cardiovascular disease. Kidney disease is also a common cause and a common complication of gout. In a UK study, people with gout had a 78% increased risk of developing moderate to severe kidney disease within three years of their gout diagnosis. Soberingly, a study from the Netherlands found that someone with gout has a risk of dying from cardiovascular disease almost seven times higher than a similar person without gout and nearly four times higher for cancer.

It should be said that in many individuals, their gout is brought on or made worse by being significantly overweight. Being overweight may be further complicated by a derangement of the body's metabolism called metabolic syndrome. Obesity increases the risk of a multitude of conditions, including diabetes, coronary heart disease, high blood pressure, liver disorders and many types of cancer. As a result, people with gout secondary to obesity may have a reduced life expectancy and be at risk of premature death. So, if you have developed gout and are significantly overweight, you should consider this a wake-up call to take determined action to lose weight, keep it off, and hopefully live a long and healthy life.

In many ways, if you have gout, the future is very much in your hands. By understanding the disease, working with your doctor, and making the appropriate lifestyle changes, you can maximise your chances of living a long and healthy life. If you try to ignore it and not make any changes, your future could be quite different.

Chapter 22

What is it like to live with gout?

Let's not mince our words; living with poorly controlled gout can be miserable. The pain of a gout attack is exquisite, and there may be constant joint pain in between attacks. It can be hard simply to do normal daily activities, leaving people dependent on family members or others, and relationships can suffer. People with gout complain that their lives have changed and their youth and health have been taken.

The pain of an acute gout attack can be so severe that it is difficult to think about anything else. Often the person enduring the pain doesn't want to do anything, doesn't want to be around anyone, and doesn't even want to eat. Normal daily activities can be difficult or impossible during an attack of gout. Just getting out of bed can be impossible, never mind climbing stairs, walking to the bathroom, brushing your hair, cooking, cleaning and gardening. People describe their whole life going on hold for a few days until the attack begins to settle.

The pain of an attack can make getting a full night's sleep a real challenge. Just having the bedsheets brush against an inflamed joint can be unbearable. It can be impossible to get comfortable, and the pain can be enough to have you lying awake, trying not to disturb a sleeping partner.

Relations with family and friends can become strained. An initial willingness to help may be tempered by the constant stress of having to do everything for someone else in addition to all they need to do themselves. It doesn't help if the person they are looking after has become

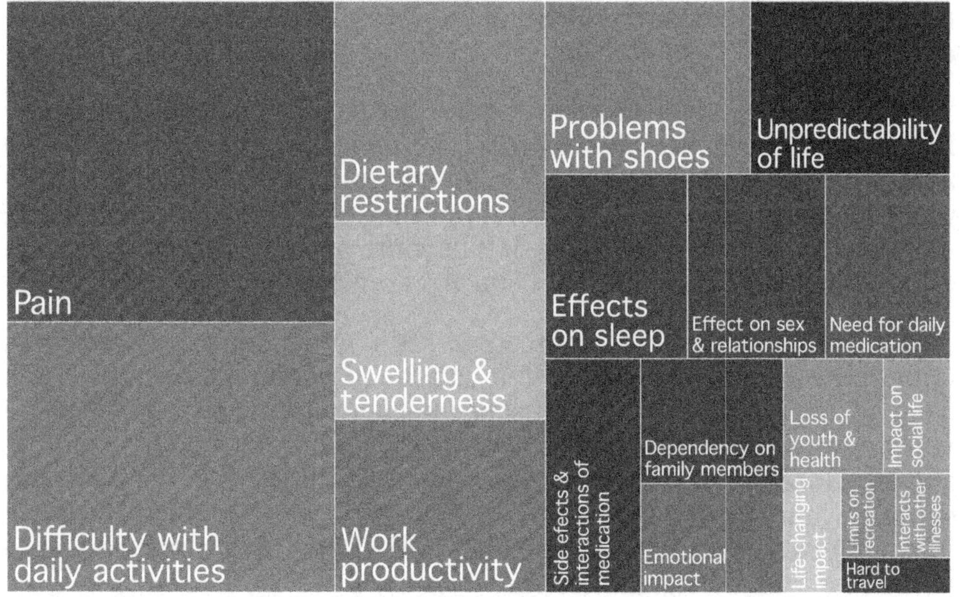

Figure 23: The impact of gout on people's lives. The size of each block represents the number of people saying this was a major issue for them. *(Adapted from "The impact of gout on patients's lives: a study of African-American and Caucasion men and women with gout" Singh, Arthritis Research & Therapy 2014, 16:R132 - used under a Creative Commons licence)*

grumpy with the pain. Sexual relations are the last thing on your mind when you're prostrated with pain. Still, the lack of intimacy can lead to a sense of separation from partners.

Apart from the practical difficulties associated with swelling and tenderness, like putting on shoes and rings, there is also a social aspect. Some people feel self-conscious about the swelling and redness, making them embarrassed to go out amongst other people.

When you can barely get about your own home, the idea of going out somewhere can seem an impossible dream. If going to the store to buy food is an insurmountable problem, how can you think about visiting friends or going to church?

A big challenge of gout is its sheer unpredictability. All the plans for the day, work, and even a vacation fly out the window when an attack strikes. It's not just your plans that are ruined; it's also the plans of those around you. At work and at home, this sudden disruption of plans can lead to frustration all around.

During a typical attack of gout, going to work is unlikely to be possible. Because of the rapid and unexpected onset of attacks, bosses who are not understanding and sympathetic can be prone to think you're just plain unreliable. It's not unheard of for people to lose their jobs because of their gout.

For many, the onset of gout may be the first experience of chronic illness, something you have to live with rather than get over. That can be a hard pill to swallow and feel like an end to the good times. It's made worse because gout can be so disabling when it strikes. Some people feel that their life has forever changed, that youth and good health are now a thing of the past. The emotional effects of this can be profound.

The dietary restrictions that come with gout can be a source of unhappiness and confusion. Often, it's the food one most enjoys – red meat, alcohol, seafood – that must be forsaken. During an attack, people may find their appetite deserts them. The pain becomes all-consuming, and food loses its attraction. But just understanding what foods you can eat and what you can't can be very confusing. It's also stressful for a family member preparing your food, worried that they'll submit you to days of agony if they get it wrong.

The need to take medication every day can be an unwelcome reminder of chronic illness, never mind the stress of actually trying to remember to take it. Additionally, there may be side effects of the medicines to deal with and the added complication of interactions with drugs being taken for other conditions.

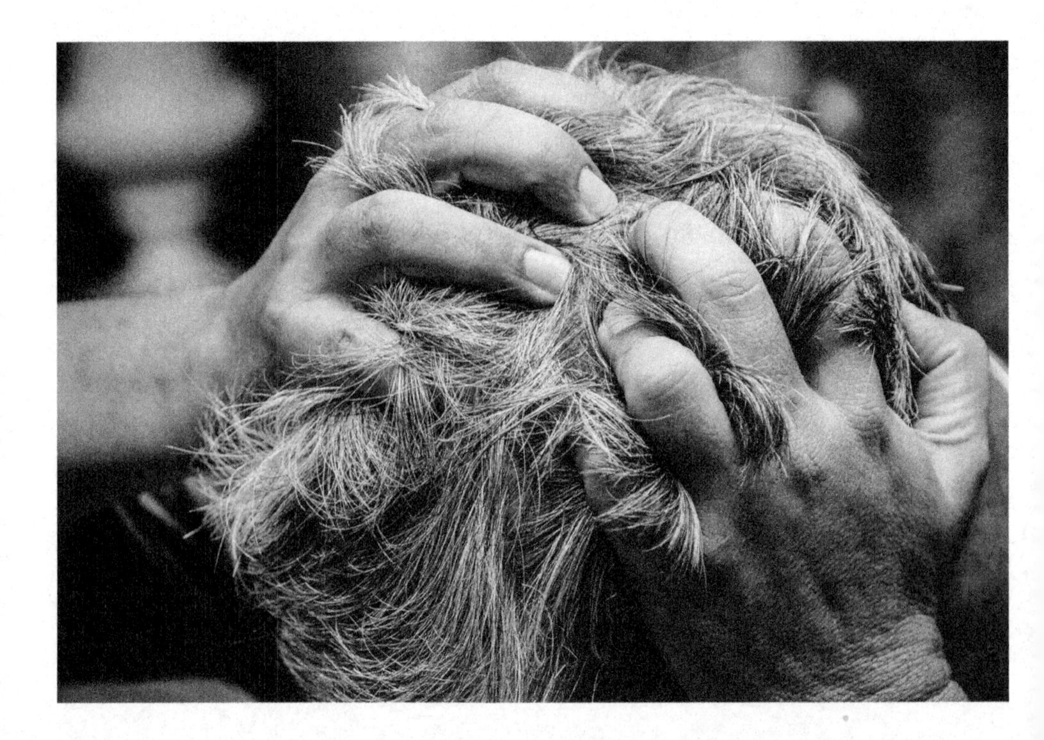

Although gout is a fairly common disease, people generally have heard of gout but know little about it. This ignorance puts added pressure on people having to explain why they suddenly have to back out of planned activities. Another major challenge is that many people believe that gout is somehow self-inflicted. Because of its caricatured reputation as the disease of gluttonous royalty, people assume that everyone with gout has brought it upon themselves by a life of over-indulgence. This can lead to a lack of compassion and understanding.

All these factors come together to affect people's emotional well-being significantly. The pain of an acute attack can be enough to make one cry. The inability to do much for yourself can make people feel helpless. While some gratefully accept the help of friends and family, others find this loss of independence intolerable. Reactions can range from depression to anger. Some say that gout attacks make them bad-tempered and mean. People looking in may not really be aware, but the effects of gout are considerably more than just a painful toe.

The good news is that the symptoms of gout can be well controlled. Life for someone with gout does not have to be miserable. However, getting to that point requires a good understanding of the disease itself and a good relationship with a diligent and knowledgeable doctor. Helping you get to that point is the reason we wrote this book.

Chapter 23

Can I pass gout on to someone else?

Gout is not an infectious disease, so you cannot pass it on to someone else on the bus or over a family dinner. However, it sometimes runs in families, demonstrating that it is possible to pass a genetic susceptibility to gout onto our children.

Variations in at least 28 genes have been identified that can affect the blood uric acid level and hence the likelihood of developing gout. The effect of each gene is relatively small but put together, it is thought that between 45% and 73% of our likelihood of getting gout comes from these inherited factors.

Our level of understanding of these genetic factors is limited, so genetic testing is not helpful at the moment; that may, however, change in the future. It is not possible, for now, to predict the likelihood of our children developing gout. However, as described elsewhere in The Handbook, the likelihood of developing gout depends not just on our genes but also on our lifestyle choices: our diet, weight, and alcohol consumption. Encouraging your children and others close to you to make healthy choices will affect their risk of developing gout as much, or more so, than any genetic factors.

Chapter 24

Which new developments should I be aware of?

In some ways, this is an exciting time for people with gout. Pharmaceutical companies, business analysts and medical technology companies have not missed the fact that rates of gout are climbing rapidly. This epidemic means a growing market for their products and so a financial driver for them to invest in new products and treatments. Here is a snapshot of some recent developments as of spring 2022.

Uric acid in coronary arteries

Recent imaging studies using dual-energy CT scans (DECT) have shown that almost 85% of people with gout have uric acid deposited in their coronary arteries. We know that higher blood uric acid levels are a risk factor for coronary heart disease and that people with gout have higher rates of cardiovascular disease. Perhaps these are related. The significance of this new finding is being investigated.

Improving treatment with an app

Staying with technological solutions, a Dutch team have completed a pilot study of a smartphone app through which people with gout can log their symptoms. Their doctor can then review the information and contact the patient to recommend changes to treatment where appropriate. Having shown that the app worked well for patients, they are now working with doctors to optimise that end of the process.

Combination therapy: pegloticase with methotrexate

One of the problems with pegloticase is that people can produce antibodies to the enzyme, reducing its effectiveness and increasing the risk of allergic reactions. Studies have shown that giving the immune-suppressing drug methotrexate at the same time as pegloticase reduces the production of antibodies and increases the number of patients who can achieve a 'complete uric acid response' from 42% to up to 90%. The company that developed pegloticase have applied for approval of this combined treatment. Combinations with other immunosuppressant drugs are also being investigated.

New drugs in development

Several brand-new medicines are being developed. SEL-212 (it hasn't got a proper drug name yet) is designed to overcome the same problem of antibodies to pegloticase. SEL-212 combines uricase with a new drug that stops the body from producing antibodies. It is in the last phase of clinical trials, but its results have not been impressive so far. Only half the patients in an earlier study maintained target uric acid levels, and its performance was not any better than pegloticase. It remains to be seen if SEL-212 will reach the market.

Tigulixostat is a new medicine that blocks xanthine oxidase – the enzyme also blocked by allopurinol and febuxostat. In a clinical trial, almost 80% of people reached their blood uric acid target of 6 mg/dL / 0.36 mmol/L. It will now go forward to more extensive trials and, if successful, will be registered for use. It is unlikely to reach the market before 2025.

ALLN-346 (again waiting for a proper name) uses an entirely new approach. It is aimed at people with gout and severe kidney impairment who have limited options for gout treatment. It works by breaking down urate in the gut, reducing urate levels in the body as a whole. It is about to start Phase II studies, where the researchers test various doses to find the best one. Years into the future, if it works well in people with chronic kidney disease, it is likely to become available for other people with gout.

ALN-XDH has the same effects as allopurinol and febuxostat but works by blocking a different enzyme (xanthine dehydrogenase) involved in urate production. It must be given by injection into the skin. It is about to start the first clinical trials in humans, so it has a long way to go.

URC-102, AR-882, dotinurad and verinurad are four new medicines with a novel way of working. They block the action of a molecule in the kidney, which reabsorbs urate from the urine. More urate passes into the urine, and less remains in the body. They are in the early stages of human trials for gout.

Effects of the gut microbiome

In an entirely new avenue of investigation, researchers found significant differences in the gut microbiome (the bacteria and other organisms that live in our guts) between men with gout and men without gout. They suggested how the differences might lead to higher uric acid levels in the blood. The field of microbiome research is still in its infancy, so there's no telling yet where this might lead in terms of new treatments. Still, it is undoubtedly a fascinating area.

As you can see, the rapid growth in the number of gout cases has led to renewed interest in developing new investigations and treatments for gout. Drug development, in particular, is a long process as vast amounts of work must be done to demonstrate to the medicines regulators that a new medicine is safe and offers benefits over existing treatments. Some of the medicines described here will not make it, but new drugs are on their way.

Chapter 25

Other crystal diseases that affect joints

Gout is the most common condition in which crystals cause pain and inflammation in joints, but it is not the only one. In this next section, we will look at one other: pseudogout. Pseudogout can mimic an attack of gout but the crystals can be distinguished under the microscope by their shape and how they look under polarised light.

Chapter 26

Pseudogout in a nutshell

You can use this chapter as a quick overview of pseudogout for yourself or for family members who want to know the basics without reading the whole section.

Pseudogout is a type of arthritis that occurs when crystals of a chemical called calcium pyrophosphate dihydrate (CPPD) form in joints. It can affect various joints, including the toes, wrists, pubic bones, and spinal joints, but the knees are the most frequently affected. It may occur in combination with osteoarthritis.

Pseudogout can cause symptoms ranging from mild intermittent or persistent aching in the affected joints to a rapid onset of pain, redness and swelling in one or more joints like gout, but usually not as severe.

Someone whose pseudogout is characterised by acute attacks may get several episodes a year. Usually, the attacks settle in a few days. In time, persistent joint aching in between attacks may occur. In long-standing disease, joint surfaces can become damaged, leading to permanent joint deformity.

The treatment of pseudogout is mostly the treatment of symptoms. Mild joint symptoms can be treated with paracetamol/acetaminophen or low doses of non-steroidal anti-inflammatory drugs (NSAIDs). Painful attacks of pseudogout are treated with higher doses of NSAIDs, with colchicine or with steroids.

For people who have frequent and painful attacks of pseudogout, a regular, ongoing dose of colchicine may reduce the frequency of attacks.

Unlike in gout, there are no treatments to lower the amount of CPPD in the body and dissolve the crystals.

Chapter 27

What is pseudogout?

Pseudogout is caused by crystals of a different chemical from those causing gout. In pseudogout, the crystals causing the problems are composed of calcium pyrophosphate dihydrate. (Gout is caused by urate crystals).

Many of us develop calcium pyrophosphate crystals in our joint cartilages and ligaments as we age. In most people, this causes no symptoms. These crystals commonly form in the knees, hands, wrists, spine, and pubic bone joints. If the crystals do cause symptoms, these can range from mild chronic arthritis pains to an acute attack that mimics gout.

This spectrum of pseudogout can be broken down into four categories:

1. CPPD crystal deposition with no symptoms
   Typically, this is found by accident when X rays are taken.

2. Acute pseudogout (also called acute CPP crystal arthritis)
   These are the rapid onset, short-lived episodes of painful joints that gave the disease its name because they are very similar to gout attacks.

3. Chronic pseudogout (also called chronic CPP crystal inflammatory arthritis)
   In this form, the joint pains are continuous.

4. Osteoarthritis with CPPD crystals
   This is when a joint with typical osteoarthritis changes also contains CPPD crystals.

Asymptomatic CPPD	Acute Pseudogout	Chronic Pseudogout	Osteoarthritis with CPPD
Crystals of CPPD are preset in cartilage & other tissues, but cause no symptoms.	*CPPD crystals in joints cause attacks of pain and swelling.*	*Chronic arthritis causes persistent joint pains.*	*Osteoarthritis with CPPD crystals in the joints. Persistent joint pains.*

Figure 24: The four types of pseudogout

Many people with pseudogout never get diagnosed. People with acute attacks will usually get medical attention as their pain can be severe. However, doctors often diagnose their attack as gout. The correct diagnosis will only be made if joint fluid is examined under a microscope. Though this is supposed to happen, most people don't have their joint fluid examined (see page 45).

Pseudogout may affect the big toe, but it is more likely to affect larger joints, especially the knee. Usually, the pain is not as severe as that of gout.

In someone who gets intermittent attacks of pseudogout, the period between episodes can be symptom-free, although there may be continuing mild pain in multiple joints. Over the long term, worsening arthritis and permanent damage to the joints may occur.

Those people with ongoing joint pains are typically treated for their symptoms without a specific diagnosis being made.

The term pseudogout may be on its way out. Experts feel it is more helpful to use terminology that describes what the disease is actually due to rather than what it mimics. The alternative names are given in the list above.

Chapter 28

What causes pseudogout?

In pseudogout, the crystals that damage the joints are of a chemical called calcium pyrophosphate dihydrate. Since that is such a mouthful, let's call it CPPD.

Pyrophosphate molecules are widespread in the body. They are involved in many chemical reactions, including the transport of energy. It has been estimated that several kilograms of pyrophosphate are involved in reactions around the body each day. However, when pyrophosphate combines with calcium to form CPPD, the new molecule is poorly soluble, and so forms crystals.

In some people, the crystals cause no problems and are found by accident on X-rays – or indeed never found at all. In other people, they cause inflammation. This inflammation leads to pain, swelling and fluid in the joint.

Unlike in gout, it is not fully understood why CPPD crystals cause problems in some people and not others. These crystals become more common as we get older and may be associated with injuries and sometimes with joint surgery, so it is thought that degenerative (wear and tear) changes in the tissues may be partially responsible.

Chapter 29

Who gets pseudogout, and how common is it?

In keeping with the thought that pseudogout is partially brought on by degenerative changes in joints and other connective tissues, it gets more common as we get older. Evidence of crystal deposits in cartilage is seen on X-ray in around 1 in 22 (4.5%) people aged 40. This rises to 1 in 5 (20%) in those over 80. In most, this causes no problems, but some people develop symptoms, usually those aged sixty and above. The risk of pseudogout appears to more than double every decade after 45 years old. Unlike gout, which is more common in men, pseudogout affects men and women equally.

Joint injuries and joint surgery, which can promote degenerative changes, also seem to increase the likelihood of getting pseudogout. In one study, joint injuries increased the risk five-fold.

Some cases run in families, implying that it can be passed on through one or more abnormal genes. In such cases, it is passed on in a dominant fashion. If either parent has the abnormal gene, the children will all get this gene and develop pseudogout. In some families, symptoms start in the 50s or 60s, but in others, there is earlier onset, usually by forty.

Certain metabolic diseases can also increase the risk of getting pseudogout. These include:

- Overactivity of the parathyroid glands.
    - ◊ The hormones produced by these small glands in the neck regulate calcium levels in the body.
    - ◊ Someone with an overactive parathyroid gland is about three times more likely to develop pseudogout.
- The iron storage disease haemochromatosis.
    - ◊ High levels of iron in the body due to this condition can cause arthritis, diabetes, liver problems and heart failure.
- Other conditions that cause low blood magnesium or phosphate.

Taking certain diuretics (water tablets), used to treat high blood pressure and fluid retention, also seems to increase the risk of pseudogout up to two-fold. The diuretics that do this include furosemide and bumetanide.

People with osteoarthritis frequently have pseudogout and vice versa. It's not clear if osteoarthritis makes pseudogout more likely, if the crystals of pseudogout contribute to osteoarthritis, or if they are simply both a consequence of ageing joints.

Chapter 30

How do I know if I have pseudogout?

Pseudogout can cause a broad range of symptoms, so it is not always easy to know that you have it.

In some cases, pseudogout can give symptoms very similar to gout: a rapid onset of pain and stiffness in a single or a small number of joints, which may be red and/or swollen. Typically, the pain is not excruciating as it usually is with gout. The pain usually reaches its worst in 6 to 24 hours.

Fever, chills and general malaise may accompany an acute attack of pseudogout. Mental confusion may be an added complication in the elderly.

An acute attack can affect a single joint or a small number. Though pseudogout can affect the big toe like gout, more commonly, larger joints are affected. The knee is most commonly involved, followed by the wrists and ankles, but any joint can be affected.

An acute attack of pseudogout is unusual in someone under sixty years old. The exception is the early-onset form that can begin in the 40s. This form typically runs in families, so it is not unexpected when it happens.

A typical attack will settle in seven to ten days if left to run its course. Sometimes it can last up to three weeks. Further attacks may occur in the same joint(s) or different ones.

In chronic pseudogout, there may be intermittent or continuing milder symptoms of aching in the affected joints. Knees, wrists and hands are commonly affected, typically on both left and right. Sometimes the structures passing through the wrist can be compressed, leading to carpal tunnel syndrome. This syndrome can cause pain in the arm or hands, pins and needles and numbness in the fingers, and sometimes a weak thumb.

People with osteoarthritis who also have CPPD crystals in the joints tend to have a somewhat different disease from those with osteoarthritis alone. Again, the knees are most affected, but the wrists and elbows are also frequently involved. Persistent joint aches are common.

Chapter 31

How will the doctor diagnose pseudogout?

In Chapter 6, we looked at the conditions that can cause pain and inflammation in one or a few joints. The doctor must weigh up the likelihood of each of those conditions based on all the available information.

The only way to make a certain diagnosis of pseudogout is to take a sample of fluid from an affected joint, as described in Chapter 8. It is important to do this for a joint that has suddenly become inflamed for the first time to make sure it is not something like a joint infection that could lead to joint damage if not properly treated.

If crystals are present in the joint fluid, they can be seen under a microscope and identified by their shape and by how they look under polarised light. In contrast to gout's needle-shaped crystals, those of CPPD in pseudogout are rhomboid or rod-shaped and appear different to gout's urate crystals under polarised light. (See next page).

White cells may be present in the joint fluid. This can be because of inflammation caused by the crystals, but it can also be a sign of infection, so the fluid is also examined and cultured in the laboratory to see if any bacteria are present.

X-rays of the affected joint are often taken. The x-rays may show patches of calcium in the joint cartilage. These are common in pseudogout, particularly in the knees, wrists, shoulders, elbows, hips, and spine. However, these patches can also be seen in people without any symptoms, in people with gout, or even with infection, so they cannot be used to prove for certain that you have pseudogout. In long-standing pseudogout, x-rays may show joint damage.

In a specialist centre, a technician may be able to see CPPD crystals in a joint using ultrasound. Ultrasound is probably better than X-rays at picking up the crystals of pseudogout in joints, but it requires expertise that is restricted to major rheumatology centres. The appearance on ultrasound is similar to that seen in gout, so it is no substitute for looking for crystals in joint fluid.

Unlike in gout, there are no blood tests that can usefully measure the amount of the CPPD chemical that forms crystals and leads to symptoms.

The diagnosis of pseudogout is not easy to make because a) pseudogout can mimic many other causes of joint discomfort, b) X-rays and ultrasound appearances are not distinctive for pseudogout, and c) there are no helpful blood tests. Examining crystals from an affected joint is the only way to make the diagnosis with certainty.

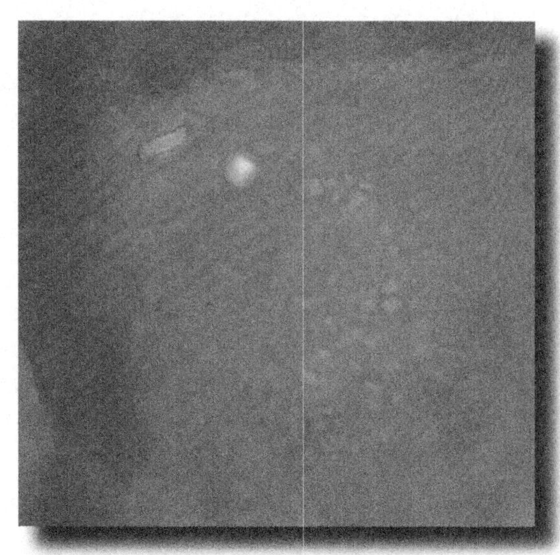

Figure 25: CPPD crystals in joint fluid, appearing blue and white under polarized light. You can see how they differ from the urate crystals of gout shown below.

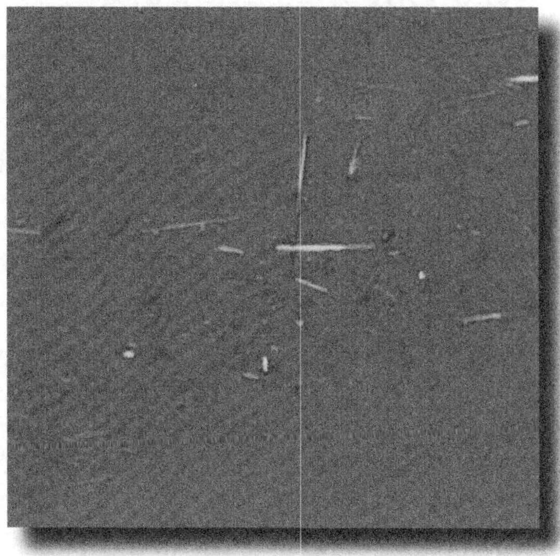

Figure 26: The needle-shaped crystals of urate that cause gout.

Chapter 32

How is pseudogout treated?

Treatment of an acute attack

Pseudogout is, in many ways, the poor relation of gout. It has been studied far less, and there is very little guidance from well-conducted clinical trials as to what is the best treatment. The treatment guidelines that have been published rely more on the experience of experts than on hard data from good studies.

A gout-like flare-up of pseudogout, with pain and perhaps swelling of a joint, is treated the same way as an attack of gout.

Most commonly, a **non-steroidal anti-inflammatory drug (NSAID)** is used to treat a flare-up of pseudogout at the same doses used to treat gout. NSAIDs are usually effective, bringing pain relief within a few hours. NSAIDs are widely used and without problems in most people but may cause gastrointestinal irritation or bleeding, fluid retention, or affect the kidneys. They may also increase the risk of a heart attack.

The elderly, those with previous stomach or duodenal ulcers, those with impairment of kidney function, and people who are dehydrated are at increased risk of side effects. You should take the lowest dose that is effective and not take more than one NSAID at a time. NSAIDs are present in many over the counter medicines, so ask a doctor or pharmacist if in doubt. The exception to this rule is low-dose aspirin being taken for its anti-platelet effect to prevent a heart attack or stroke. NSAIDs should be taken with a full glass of water with or immediately after a meal to reduce the risk of stomach irritation. NSAIDs are discussed in more detail in Chapter 9 and Chapter 13.

It is primarily the elderly who get pseudogout, and the elderly are at a higher risk of side effects from NSAIDs. They also often have other conditions that further increase the risk of side effects, so using NSAIDs to treat pseudogout can be problematic.

An alternative to NSAIDs is **colchicine**. A dose of 1 or 1.2 mg is taken immediately, followed by another 0.5 or 0.6 mg dose on day one. In the following days, 0.5 or 0.6 mg is taken two or three times daily during the acute attack. (Different strength tablets are available in different countries, hence the 0.5 or 0.6 mg). Pain relief usually occurs in 12 to 24 hours. To be effective, colchicine must be given as early as possible in an attack, ideally within 12 to 24 hours of the attack starting. If taken within a few hours, colchicine can stop an attack before it really gets started. Wait until a couple of days after the attack has begun, though, and it is much less effective. For this reason, if your attacks are treated with colchicine, you should keep a starter pack with you. Colchicine is discussed in more detail in Chapter 9 and Chapter 13.

Steroids are frequently used to treat pseudogout. One of the reasons is that NSAIDs and colchicine can have unacceptable side effects in the elderly. Short courses of steroids are generally safer, and they work well. Steroids may be given either as tablets (usually prednisolone or prednisone) or by injection.

A particularly effective treatment for an attack of pseudogout is to drain the fluid from the joint and then use the same needle to inject steroids into the joint. It is essential to ensure there is no joint infection before using this treatment.

Resting the affected joint and using ice packs around it can both help to relieve the pain of an acute attack.

Prevention of recurrent attacks

After a first attack of pseudogout, some people may have further attacks, while others will have no more. Whether you take medication to prevent further flare-ups will depend on the frequency and severity of those attacks.

The frequency of further attacks may be reduced by taking **colchicine** 0.5 or 0.6 mg twice daily. The use of colchicine is discussed further in Chapter 9 and Chapter 13.

Whether **non-steroidal anti-inflammatory drugs (NSAIDs)** taken long term prevent further pseudogout attacks has not been adequately investigated. Given that most people with pseudogout are elderly, the long-term use of NSAIDs comes with significant safety concerns. Particular worries are kidney damage, heart attacks, heart failure, and stomach ulcers. Under these circumstances, using NSAIDs to prevent pseudogout attacks may not be a great idea.

Unlike for gout, there are no treatments to reduce the level of CPPD in the body to prevent further attacks.

Treatment of ongoing joint symptoms

People with the persistent form of pseudogout, now often called chronic CPP crystal inflammatory arthritis, are usually treated with **non-steroidal anti-inflammatory drugs (NSAIDs).** The lowest effective dose should be used, but in the elderly, this may still cause unacceptable side effects. The risk of stomach and duodenal ulcers may be reduced by giving a drug that blocks the production of stomach acid at the same time. NSAIDs are discussed in more detail in Chapter 9 and Chapter 13.

One small study investigated the use of **colchicine** to treat osteoarthritis with CPPD crystals. In this study, 0.5 mg of colchicine twice daily was effective at controlling joint pain and did not cause significant side effects. The use of colchicine to treat chronic pseudogout has not been properly studied.

A few small studies have looked at three potential treatments for chronic pseudogout.

- The antimalarial drug **hydroxychloroquine** (also used to treat rheumatoid arthritis) improved symptoms in 85% of study participants within two months. This study was very small but showed promise. However, it was a long time ago (1997), and the use of hydroxychloroquine for pseudogout has not been further investigated.

- Although no proper studies have been done, a few patients with chronic pseudogout have been treated with **anakinra**, which stops inflammation by interfering with a pro-inflammatory chemical in the body. Most of these patients have had a good response to the treatment. Because anakinra has to be given by injection, is expensive, and comes with the risk of severe infections, it is recommended only for people whose chronic pseudogout causes them a lot of pain or disability and who can't be treated with other medicines.

- Destroying the lining of the joint with **radiation** sounds over the top, but in one study, this led to less pain, stiffness, tenderness and fluid in the treated knees. The researchers injected the knees with radioactive yttrium-90 and steroids for this study. This treatment is used occasionally for people with chronic pseudogout who have recurrent bleeding into the joint.
- Low doses of the immune-suppressant drug **methotrexate** (5 – 10 mg/week) gave an excellent result in terms of reducing pain, swelling and the frequency of flare-ups in one study. No significant side effects were reported. However, another group of researchers repeated this study and found that methotrexate didn't work.

These four treatments are all very much experimental in the treatment of pseudogout. Large, well-designed studies would need to be done to see if they are useful and safe to use routinely.

Chapter 33

What questions should I ask the doctor about my diagnosis and initial treatment?

This book aims to provide you with information and understanding so that you can talk with confidence to your doctor and understand the decisions they make. The questions suggested here are meant as openings for discussion so that you can understand and be involved in the decisions made about your health. To participate in those discussions, you should have read the appropriate sections in the Handbook.

The diagnosis of pseudogout is often not as straightforward as it is for gout. The symptoms may more closely resemble various other conditions, including the very common osteoarthritis, which is simply due to wear and tear on the joints.

Since there are no specific treatments required for pseudogout, the priority is to rule out other conditions that do not require specific treatment, especially those that can cause lasting damage if untreated.

The most important thing to exclude is a joint infection for someone with a first attack of sudden onset of painful, inflamed joints. Your doctor may consider just treating it as a case of gout. That will work out fine most of the time, as non-steroidal anti-inflammatory drugs (NSAIDs) will treat the symptoms of joint pain and inflammation whatever the course. However, this approach would miss cases of joint infection, which may go on to cause joint damage, and would not give a definitive diagnosis of gout or pseudogout, which is needed to guide future treatment. Therefore, if your doctor suggests treating you without confirming the diagnosis for certain, it would be appropriate to ask: "Can you be sure of the diagnosis? Would it be helpful to examine some joint fluid to make sure it's not a joint infection and see which type of crystal is present?"

Chapter 34

How should my progress be monitored?

Compared to gout, the treatment of pseudogout is much less complicated. Far fewer drugs are available, and it is not possible to reduce or even monitor blood levels of CPPD. Monitoring progress is down to making sure pain in acute atacks is well controlled and ensuring that recurrent attacks are reduced by colchicine if necessary.

Acute attacks

In an acute attack of pseudogout, the most important considerations are controlling the pain and making sure there's nothing else going on.

If pain control is not adequate, then either an increase in dose or a change in medication should be considered.

Pseudogout attacks usually settle in a few days. If an attack fails to resolve or feels significantly different from previous episodes, then further investigations may be necessary to make sure that the symptoms really are due to gout and only gout.

Reducing the frequency of attacks

After the first attack of pseudogout, it is important to note how often further attacks occur. There may be no more or very few with a long time in between attacks. If attacks happen more than once a year, your doctor may decide to put you on daily preventative treatment with colchicine.

Monitoring the side-effects of medication

Certain drugs given for pseudogout can cause side-effects that may be picked up early and effectively through blood tests. How often these tests should be done depends very much on your individual circumstances, other medical conditions you may have, and any other medicines you may be taking. Table 16 lists the normally recommended tests for medicines taken for gout

	Kidney tests	Liver tests	Blood count
Colchicine	✓	✓	✓
NSAIDs	✓		✓
Prednisolone			

Table 16: Recommended blood tests for pseudogoutgout medicines – frequency and timing of tests depends on many things. Talk to your doctor to find out how often you should have these tests.

Chapter 35

What questions should I ask the doctor at follow up visits?

This book aims to provide you with information and understanding so that you can talk with confidence to your doctor and understand the decisions they make. The questions suggested here are meant as openings for discussion so that you can understand and be involved in the decisions made about your health. To participate in those discussions, you should have read the appropriate sections in the Handbook.

Once a firm diagnosis of pseudogout has been made by examining crystals from the fluid of an affected joint, the critical issue becomes the prevention of future attacks and joint damage. Some people will have further attacks while others will not. If you have frequent and painful attacks that interfere with your life, it would be reasonable to ask your doctor, "Do you think I should be taking colchicine to prevent further attacks?"

Chapter 36

What can I do for myself?

In addition to taking any medication prescribed by your doctor, there are measures you can take yourself to help with your pseudogout.

In an acute attack, the affected joint should be rested. Ice packs can help reduce pain and swelling. If necessary, you can splint the painful joint.

A commercial splint is the easiest and most effective way to immobilize knees and wrists. Elbows and shoulders can be rested by putting the arm in a sling. If you are improvising yourself at home, be careful that a splint is not tied on too tightly and impairing the circulation. Ensure also that the splint does not rub on the skin and cause abrasions.

All forms of arthritis are made worse if you are overweight as this puts a higher load on the joint. If you are overweight, take the time to adjust your diet and activities so that you can get down to a healthier weight. It will have benefits way beyond helping with your pseudogout.

Walking, cycling and especially swimming are recommended for people with pseudogout as ways to maintain joint flexibility without putting too much pressure on the joints. It is important to get up and about as soon as possible as an attack begins to settle.

Unlike for gout, there are no specific foods that help or make pseudogout worse.

Chapter 37

Under what circumstances should I see my doctor immediately?

After the first one or two attacks of pseudogout, you will likely recognise subsequent attacks without difficulty, and you will have been advised by your doctor on what medication to take for an attack. However, you should see your doctor if an attack feels very different to the ones you've had before or if it is not settling down within a few days. Just because you have gout doesn't mean you can't get inflamed joints from other causes, including bacterial joint infections.

Non-steroidal anti-inflammatory drugs (NSAIDs) have been associated with an increased risk of cardiovascular disease. If you develop chest pain or tightness, you should contact your doctor immediately or go to the hospital emergency department. You could be having a heart attack.

If you are taking non-steroidal anti-inflammatory drugs and develop severe indigestion, vomit blood or 'coffee grounds', or pass black stools, you should contact your doctor immediately or go to the hospital emergency department. You could be bleeding from stomach inflammation or an ulcer caused by the drugs.

A small number of people taking colchicine have developed serious liver inflammation (hepatitis). You should see your doctor if you develop jaundice: yellowing of the skin and whites of the eyes and passing dark urine.

A very rare side effect of colchicine is suppression of the bone marrow. Once this becomes severe, the symptoms are fever, sore throat, bruising and bleeding. You should see your doctor immediately if you develop these symptoms.

Symptom	May be due to
Severe indigestion, vomiting blood or 'coffee-grounds' or passing black stools	Bleeding from stomach inflammation or ulcer
An attack that isn't settling down in a few days	A joint infection
An attack that feels quite different from previous attacks	A joint infection
Chest pain or tightness, sweating and shortness of breath	A heart attack
Yellowing of the skin and eyes and passing dark urine	Jaundice from liver inflammation
Fever, sore throat, bruising and bleeding	Bone marrow suppression

Table 17: Contact your doctor if you have any of these symptoms.

Chapter 38

Can I pass on pseudogout to someone else?

As with gout, pseudogout is not infectious. You cannot pass it on to someone else through contact. Sometimes, but by no means always, pseudogout runs in families, which shows that it can be passed on through the genes we give to our children. In these cases of inherited pseudogout it is typically passed on as a dominant gene. This means that if either parent has this form of pseudogout it will be passed on to their children.

Again, only a proportion of cases of pseudogout are inherited. In other cases it does not seem to be passed from parents to their children.

Chapter 39

What is the long-term outlook with pseudogout?

Even without treatment, individual flare-ups of pseudogout will settle down within one to three weeks. As time goes by, some people with pseudogout will develop persistent aching in the affected joints. This is more common in older people, and most of us develop aching in a few joints as we get older, so it might not seem out of the ordinary.

For most people with osteoarthritis-related pseudogout, disease progression occurs slowly, if at all. If gradual worsening of joint symptoms does occur, it's usually in the knees, hips or shoulders.

A small proportion of people with pseudogout may develop more severe damage to the joints, which can eventually become deformed. This occurs mainly in elderly women and can be very painful. Sometimes bleeding into the joints occurs.

Chapter 40

Is physiotherapy useful for gout and pseudogout?

Physiotherapy (physical therapy) can undoubtedly play a valuable role in managing gout and pseudogout.

During acute attacks, a physiotherapist will be able to help with splinting the affected joint.

The physiotherapist will assess your mobility between attacks and see if any devices such as walking sticks or walking frames are needed. They can also provide therapy and exercises to maintain full movement at the joints and improve muscle strength to ensure your arms and legs maintain full function.

Gout and especially pseudogout occur most often in older adults. In this age group, being 'off your legs' for a week or two can have serious consequences. An episode of immobility due to a gout attack can easily lead to long term reduced mobility. A physiotherapist with a program of exercises and encouragement can quickly ensure that you get back to full functioning.

Chapter 41

Complementary and alternative treatments

Many people's gout is not as well controlled as they would like on conventional medicine, and they worry about the potential side effects of conventional treatments. Hence there is considerable interest in alternative or complementary therapies for gout. After spending a few days reviewing the many recommendations on gout-related websites and forums, we were left unsurprised that many people are confused about which to consider trying. The difficulty with alternative treatments is that they have never been subjected to the intense, formal scrutiny and studies required to get conventional drugs licenced. Because of this, there is insufficient evidence to be clear about their usefulness and safety. Here is our best attempt to make sense of it all.

Water: It may seem strange to see plain old water on this list of non-medicinal treatments for gout, but in fact, increasing your water consumption can be extremely helpful. Drinking more water means that your kidneys must excrete it, and the urate is excreted with it. Gout forms because urate is poorly soluble in water, so the more water passes through the body, the more urate can be dissolved and carried away. There have been hardly any formal studies of the relationship between water intake and gout. Still, one study did show that men drinking more than 3 litres of water per day and women drinking more than 2.2 litres were 60% less likely to have a high uric acid level (6 mg/dL

(0.36 mmol/l)). Not having a high uric acid means fewer gout attacks and fewer complications.

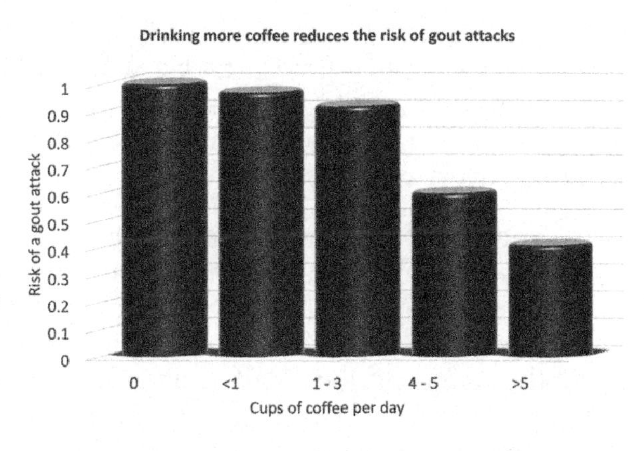

Figure 27: Dinking more coffee reduces the risk of gout attacks.

Coffee: Here's some news that will make many people happy: drinking more coffee reduces your chances of having gout attacks. As you can see from the graph, the effect seems to really kick in when you drink four or more cups of coffee each day.

The caffeine in coffee appears to inhibit xanthine oxidase, the enzyme in the body that produces uric acid. This is a likely mechanism by which coffee reduces the risk of gout, and blood uric acid levels do decrease with increased coffee consumption. Coffee also contains a chemical called chlorogenic acid, a potent antioxidant and may help reduce inflammation.

Some other effects of coffee diminish over time, and no long-term studies have investigated the reduction in gout attacks with coffee, so the effect may get less with continued coffee consumption.

A small protective effect was seen with decaffeinated coffee, but it is much less, and sadly for us tea drinkers, no protective effect has been shown with tea.

Omega-3 polyunsaturated fatty acids: These are mainly obtained from oily fish such as mackerel, salmon, herring, sardines and oysters, or as a supplement. Researchers from Boston asked more than 700 gout patients about their consumption of oily fish or omega-3 supplements when they were well and when they had gout attacks. They found that eating oily fish gave around 25% protection against gout attacks, whereas taking omega-3 supplements had no protective effect.

Cherries: It is thought that about a quarter of people with gout use cherries or a cherry product (cherry extract or cherry juice) as an alternative or complementary treatment. Cherries contain various beneficial chemicals, including vitamins A, C and E, and both anthocyanins and quercetin, which both have antioxidant and anti-inflammatory properties. The amounts present vary inconsistently between sweet and sour cherries making it hard to say if sweet or sour cherries are a better choice.

In one large, well-designed study, eating cherries was associated with a 35% lower risk of gout attacks, while taking cherry extracts led to a 45% reduction in attacks. Cherry products taken with allopurinol led to a 75% reduction in attacks. The effects of cherries peaked at three servings every two days.

In another very small study, people taking one tablespoon of cherry juice concentrate twice a day for four months saw their gout attacks fall from five in four months to one and a half attacks over the same period. Half were attack-free after six months, including 36% on cherry juice concentrate alone without allopurinol.

There is evidence, then, that cherries have a potential role in the long-term prevention of gout attacks. To prove it beyond a reasonable doubt would require a large, high-quality study, and so far, no such trial has taken place. In the meantime, it is understandable that many people are taking cherries or cherry extract in the hope of benefit.

Turmeric: Turmeric has been used in Ayurvedic medicine for several thousand years and is thought to have anti-inflammatory properties. People vary in their ability to absorb the chemicals in turmeric, with some only absorbing 5%, so the results of studies can be variable. Side effects tend to be mild and include itching and diarrhoea at high doses.

In a study of 39 people with raised blood uric acid levels, after eight weeks of taking 500mg curcumin capsules (an extract of turmeric) twice daily, uric acid levels had fallen by almost 7%. However, levels had also dropped by 5% in those taking dummy capsules. There was no statistical difference between the two groups. It is common in studies for people taking dummy pills to experience benefits (the so-called placebo effect). This occurs because they a) believe they will see benefits, b) pay increased attention to diet and other lifestyle factors, and c) get better medical care from seeing a doctor regularly for the study assessments.

In another study of 19 people using a commercial preparation of curcumin (Flexofytol) designed to be better absorbed from the gut, 17 of those 19 experienced relief from the symptoms of an acute attack comparable to non-steroidal anti-inflammatory drugs, as did 20 of 23 later patients not included in the study. Eleven of the 19 decided to continue taking the capsules to prevent future attacks. This study did not use dummy pills for comparison, so it's impossible to say how much of the effect was due to the placebo effect.

Based on the evidence, it's not clear if turmeric is useful in treating gout, but it is worth exploring further. A well-conducted, properly designed study is needed to answer the question.

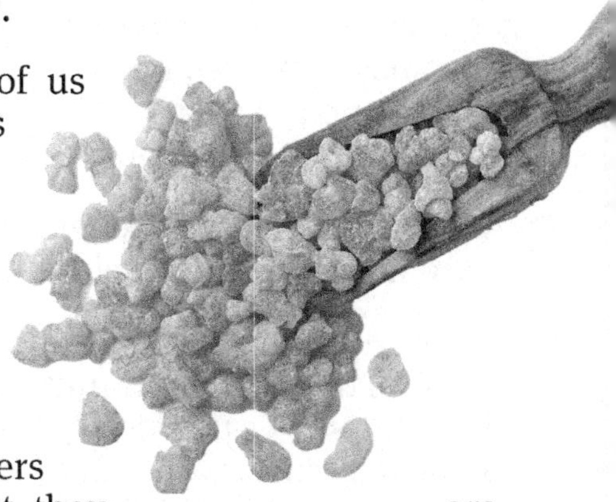

Boswellia: Better known to many of us as frankincense, the resin from this tree has been demonstrated to have anti-inflammatory and pain-killing properties. In small studies of people with knee osteoarthritis, Boswellia was significantly better than dummy tablets at reducing pain and improving knee function and even led to X-ray improvements in the joint. Reviewers of these studies have concluded that they are not of good enough quality to justify recommendations for the use of Boswellia. However, they were promising enough that further large, well-designed studies should be conducted to investigate the usefulness of Boswellia. The use of Boswellia in gout has not been studied.

Rosemary: We could not identify any studies investigating the effect of rosemary in people with gout. However, rosemary has been shown to add to the pain-killing effects of some non-steroidal anti-inflammatory drugs, so it may be helpful if taken in conjunction with these.

Vitamin C: Vitamin C is commonly recommended as a supplement for people with gout because it has been shown to increase the excretion of urate by the kidneys. Several studies have shown that higher levels of vitamin C in the blood are associated with a lower blood uric acid level. However, there is no clear evidence that taking vitamin C supplements reduces the frequency or severity of recurrent gout attacks. In a recent, thorough review of all the evidence, researchers concluded that the best advice was to recommend a diet rich in fruits and vegetables and low in meat rather than the use of vitamin C supplements.

Vitamin C is generally regarded as safe, though it can cause diarrhoea at higher doses.

Apple cider vinegar: Although apple cider vinegar is often recommended for treating gout, there is no substantial evidence that it works. In one very small study of just 39 people, those who took apple cider vinegar in addition to a restricted-calorie diet lost more weight and had less of an appetite than those who only had the restricted calorie diet. Since weight loss can be beneficial in reducing the risk of recurrent gout attacks, this could be beneficial, but we could not find any studies that looked at the effectiveness of apple cider vinegar in preventing gout attacks directly. In one laboratory study, lab-made red-koji vinegar contained two chemicals that reduce xanthine oxidase activity, the enzyme that produces uric acid in the body. However, no studies have looked at whether this happens in the body or has any effect in gout. It's also unclear if the same chemicals are present in commercially bought vinegar.

Apple cider vinegar is generally considered safe, though its high acidity could damage tooth enamel and cause indigestion, acid reflux and nausea.

Ginger: Ginger is often prescribed in Eastern medical traditions to treat gout. It is said to have anti-inflammatory properties. One study conducted in Pakistan shows promising results. Almost all patients in the study had a marked decrease in their blood uric acid levels and gout symptoms after 18 weeks of treatment. However, the researchers did not use ginger alone; rather, a herbal medicine called Gouticin, which contains extracts from six medicinal plants, including Colchicum autumnale, the plant from which colchicine is extracted. It is, therefore, impossible to work out which of the ingredients contributed to the effects.

In a study in rats, a ginger extract lowered uric acid levels in animals with artificially induced high uric acid levels but did nothing for normal rats, whereas allopurinol reduced uric acid in both groups.

Based on these findings, there is no clear evidence that ginger is of use in treating gout, though further studies may be warranted.

Lemons: In a small, unreviewed, 2015 pilot study, 75 rheumatology patients, some of whom had gout, were asked to drink the juice of two freshly squeezed lemons in two litres of water each day for six weeks. At the end of that period, blood uric acid levels had fallen by an average of between 1.0 and 1.6 mg/dL, a fall that could be significant in treating gout.

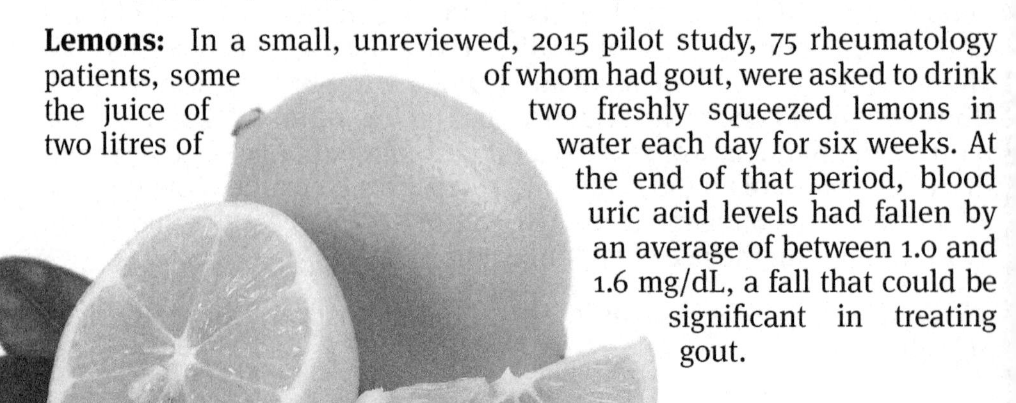

On the face of it, this looks great. However, there should have been a comparison group who drank two litres of water a day without the lemon juice to see if it was just the two litres of extra water per day that made the difference. There have been no follow up studies published. So, using lemon juice to treat gout remains an intriguing but unproven idea.

Garlic: Gout-related web articles frequently recommend garlic as a treatment for gout, claiming that it lowers blood uric acid levels and reduces inflammation. We have not been able to find any studies testing whether garlic lowers blood uric acid levels, so this seems to be pure conjecture.

Several laboratory studies attest to the anti-inflammatory effects of garlic, particularly aged garlic extract, and trials in humans show that this can benefit some diseases. Garlic has been shown to offer some benefits in treating knee osteoarthritis in overweight women, but we could not find any studies of garlic being used to treat gout.

There is currently no clear evidence that garlic is beneficial in treating gout.

Skimmed milk powder enriched with glycomacropeptides (GMP/G600): A single small study of 120 patients looked at the effectiveness of glycomacropeptides in gout. Those taking skimmed milk powder enriched with GMPs had an average of six gout episodes per year compared to eight per year for those taking plain skimmed milk powder. Reviewers considered the evidence unconvincing and said there was no evidence to recommend using GMP-enriched skimmed milk powder in gout.

Sodium bicarbonate: The belief that taking sodium bicarbonate or baking soda might be beneficial in gout comes from the fact that gout is due to an excess of uric acid (technically the uric acid salt sodium urate) and that sodium bicarbonate neutralises acids. There is no evidence that sodium bicarbonate is helpful. In fact, a study with 45 patients given sodium bicarbonate over 20 weeks showed no effect whatsoever on uric acid levels.

Bloodletting: A recent scientific review of 12 Chinese studies of bloodletting garnered much press attention. The reviewers concluded that bloodletting was safe and as effective as 'Western' medicine in gout treatment. The studies they looked at were all very small, and in 8 of the 12 studies, the amount of blood taken was tiny, less than 10ml. That's the same as a routine blood test. The studies were also flawed in that both patients and their healthcare practitioners knew which patients were being treated with bloodletting and which were not. This means there was no way to exclude the placebo effect (when patients benefit from dummy tablets or treatments) or bias from the practitioners who already believed that bloodletting was effective. Much larger, well-conducted studies would be needed to determine if there is a real benefit from bloodletting.

Others: A review of many gout-related websites and forums led to lots of other less common recommendations for alternative gout treatments, for none of which were we able to find convincing evidence that they worked. Among that list were:

Bananas and cucumbers: these are low in purines, so not bad for someone with gout, but there's no evidence of any specific anti-gout properties. **Red pepper flakes, fenugreek, carom seeds/ajwain, mustard seeds/oil:** again, there is nothing to support their usefulness in gout. **Plantain** (the plant Plantago major, often considered a weed, not the fruit related to the banana) is widely used in Chinese medicine and is said to have anti-inflammatory activity. Though scientists have suggested how it may be effective in treating gout, we have not been able to find any human studies testing its effectiveness. **Devil's Claw:** A few studies in patients with arthritis have shown conflicting results. In some, the patients felt their symptoms had improved, while there seemed to be little effect in others. None of the studies used a dummy pill to make sure the effects were real and not due to the placebo effect, and no studies have looked at people with gout. **Bromelain**, an extract from pineapple stems, is thought to have some anti-inflammatory effects. Studies in osteoarthritis have shown conflicting results. Its use in gout has not been adequately studied.

Methylsulfonylmethane (MSM): is said to have anti-inflammatory properties. In studies, MSM showed some effects in treating the pain of osteoarthritis, but these were not thought to be clinically significant. It has not been adequately studied in gout.

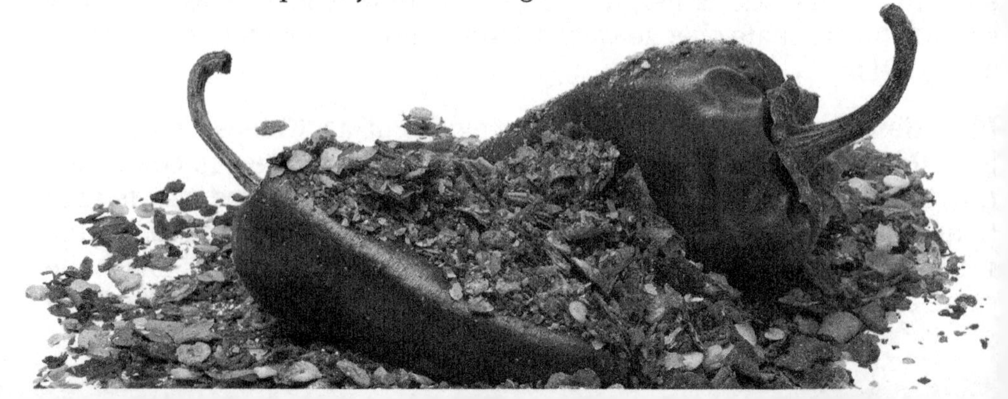

In summary

So, after all that, what are we to conclude? After careful review of the evidence, here's what we think.

Actions likely to bring significant benefits	Unproven, but possibly helpful
Drink at least 3 litres of fluids a day if you are a man, or 2.2 litres if you're a woman. Add lemon juice if you want.	Consider taking a cherry extract.
Drink at least 4 cups of coffee a day.	Consider taking supplements containing turmeric/curcumin and/or Boswellia.
Eat a diet rich in fruit and vegetables.	Consider taking rosemary supplements for pain relief in acute gout attacks.
Eat oily fish regularly.	
Eat cherries most days.	

In addition to the turmeric and rosemary mentioned above, feel free to also liven up your cooking with garlic, ginger, lemon juice, apple cider vinegar, red pepper flakes, fenugreek and mustard seeds, but we don't see enough evidence to support taking them as supplements.

You should talk to your doctor before taking herbal or other complementary medicines as they may sometimes interact with other medications you are taking or exacerbate other medical conditions you may have.

Chapter 42

Gout in history

Gout was recognised and described by the Egyptians as long ago as 2640 BC. It was described as 'the unwalkable disease' by the famous Greek physician Hippocrates. Hippocrates is well known to doctors. When we first qualify, we take the Hippocratic Oath, promising, 'First do no harm.'

Another famous Greek physician, Galen, was the first to describe tophi early in the 2nd century AD. An Anglo-Saxon manuscript from the late 9th century describes herbal remedies for gout. One of the pioneers of microscopy, Antoni van Leeuwenhoek, was the first to describe urate crystals he obtained from a tophus in 1679.

Hippocrates, Galen and the Roman senator Seneca all associated gout with overindulgence and debauchery. This way of thinking persists and is an added challenge for people coping with gout today.

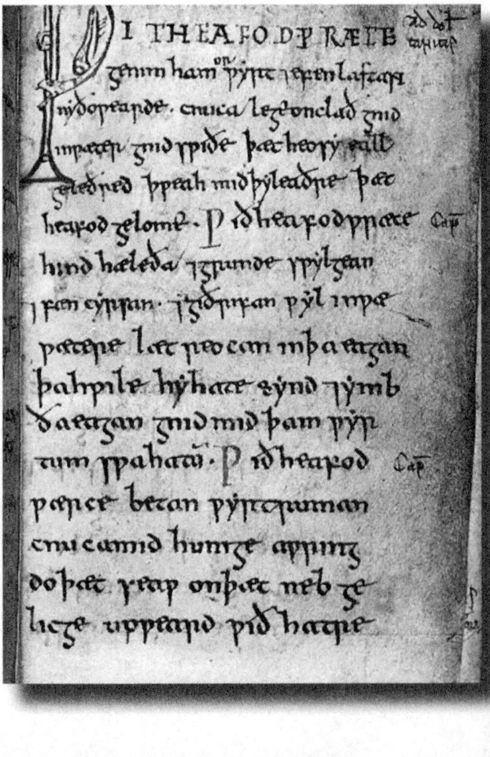

Figure 28: The Lacnunga, an Anglo-Saxon book of remedies from the late 9th century AD, describes herbal treatments for gout.

Gout has long been regarded as a disease of royalty. There may be a number of reasons for this: the most popular being that gout is a disease of dietary excess, but historically the life of our monarchs has been much more closely monitored than that of the common people, so their illnesses are more widely reported. Nevertheless, since we know that meat is a rich source of purines, their lavish diet likely contributed to the development of gout.

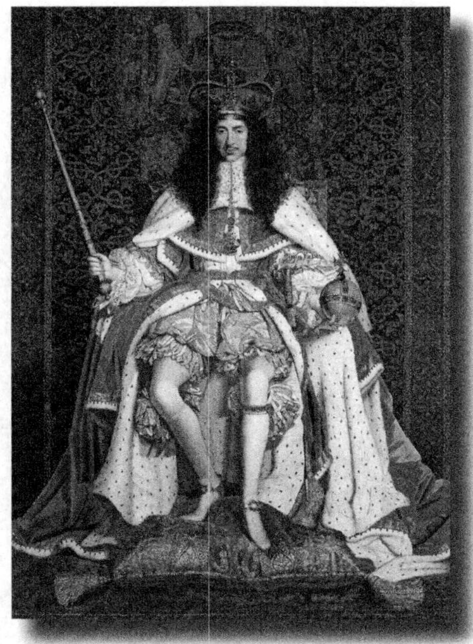

Figure 29: England's King Charles II. When gout prevented him taking the walks he loved so much, he started practicing alchemy, and that probably killed him.

England's Henry VIII usually tops the list of monarchs affected by gout, he of the eight wives. In fact, it is not certain that he suffered from gout, but certainly, in his later years, he was obese and relatively immobile. The English King James I suffered badly with both gout and kidney stones. Charles II's gout prevented him from taking the long walks he had always enjoyed. Instead, he took to his laboratory to try to distil mercury. The toxic fumes may have contributed to his death. Queen Anne was suffering from an attack of gout at her coronation. She had to be carried to Westminster Abbey in a sedan chair. In her later life, she was rendered lame by her gout. George IV was known for his vast banquets and profuse alcohol consumption even before becoming king. He was ridiculed for his obesity. Later in his reign, gout in his right arm prevented him from signing documents.

Across the English Channel, Louis XIV, the so-called Sun King and longest-reigning monarch of any sovereign country, projected the image of a healthy and virile man, but in reality, gout was just one of his many debilitating ailments. Louis XVIII, returned to the throne in the Bourbon Restoration after the French Revolution, suffered recurrent attacks of gout, and was crippled in later years by his gout and corpulence. The last king of France, Napoleon III, also suffered from gout, kidney stones, and arthritis. Frederick the Great, King of Prussia, also suffered from gout in his later years, as had his father.

Several sultans of the Ottoman dynasty had gout, beginning with Osman I, the dynasty's founder. He is said to have suffered greatly from

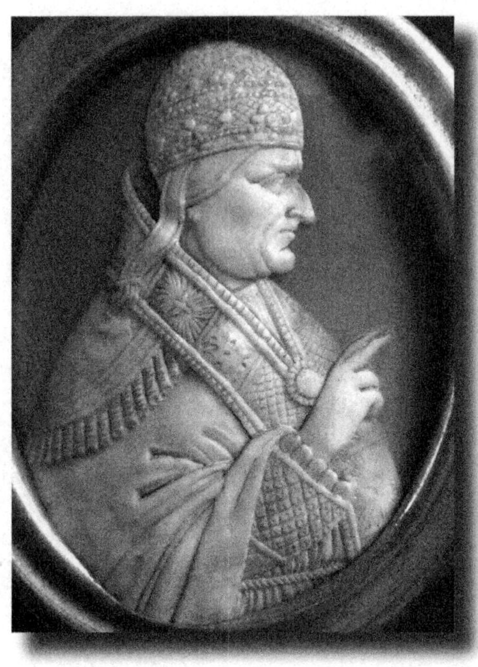

Figure 30: Pope Honorius IV was so crippled with gout that he could neither walk nor stand, and had a machine made to raise the bread and wine in his hands when he celebrated Mass.

pain in his foot which frequently stopped him from fighting in his military campaigns. After the failure of his military campaigns in Vietnam and Japan and the death of his favourite wife and chosen heir, Kublai Khan turned to food and drink. His weight ballooned, and he became grossly overweight, suffering from gout and diabetes.

The Holy Roman Emperors did not escape gout either. Conrad II, ruler of Germany, Italy and Burgundy, died of gout in 1039 in Utrecht, where his heart and bowels are buried. The rest of him was buried at Speyer Cathedral in Germany. Charles IV had gout, as did Charles V, who, during the Schmalkaldic War, was carried semi-conscious with gout from the siege of Innsbruck and barely escaped with his life. In later life, he would become crippled by his gout, as was his later successor, Charles VII.

The papacy has also seen its share of gout sufferers. Pope Honorius IV was already elderly and so crippled with gout that he could neither stand nor walk at the time of his consecration. He had to sit to celebrate mass and had a mechanical contraption constructed to raise his hands with the host. Pope Clement VIII is said to have been the first pope to drink coffee, but despite coffee's protective effects, Clement was confined to bed for much of his later life with gout. Pope Clement X, the oldest pope at the time of his

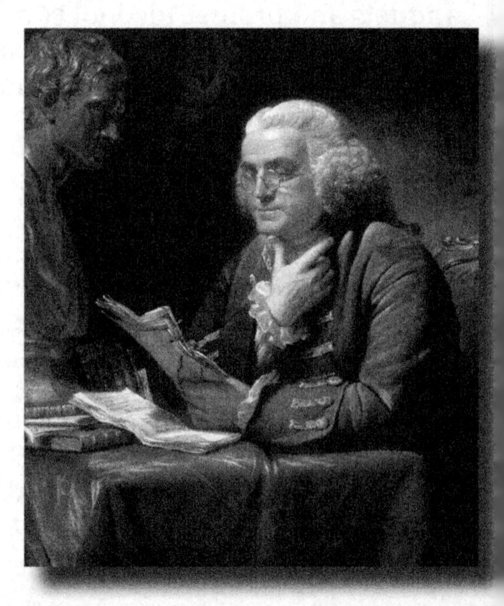

Figure 31: Benjamin Franklin, one of the Founding Fathers of the United States, was suffering so badly from a gout attack that he couldn't make it to most of the meetings to draft the US Constitution.

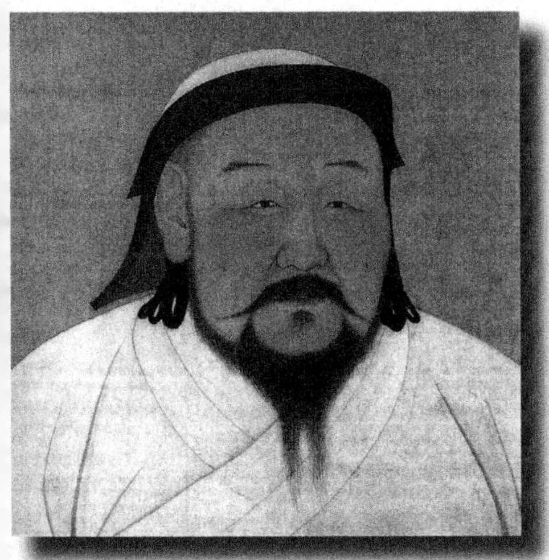

Figure 32: The great Mongol leader Kublai Khan. After military and personal losses he sought comfort in food, but found only gout.

election (seventy-nine, in case you were wondering), died in agony from gout in 1676. Clement XII, who began the construction of Rome's Trevi Fountain, also died from gout.

The political classes have also been afflicted with gout. Four British Prime Ministers are known to have had gout. William Pitt the Elder and his son William Pitt the Younger both had gout. Pitt the Elder had his first gout attack at Eton School and later was forced to leave Oxford University without completing his degree because of his gout. As Prime Minister, he had to be carried to Parliament for an important debate on the Treaty of Paris, during which he gave an impassioned three-hour speech frequently interrupted by paroxysms of pain. Pitt the Younger also suffered from gout said to have been made worse by his passion for port wine, which gained him the nickname 'the three-bottle man'. More recently, Dennis Healey and French President Jacques Chirac were said to have suffered from gout, as do Michael Heseltine and North Korea's Kim Jong-Un.

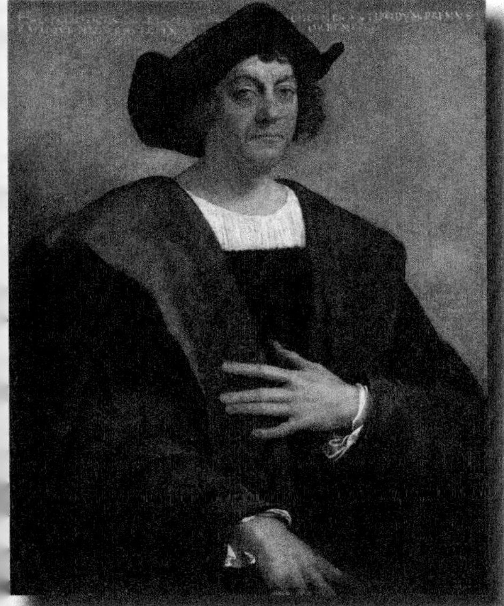

Figure 33: Christopher Columbus. On his many voyages around the world, he was plagued with gout - though a few historians think it might have been a venereal disease.

Across the Atlantic, two of the United States' Founding Fathers also had to deal with gout. Benjamin Franklin was one of the Committee of Five that drafted the Declaration of Independence. In fact, he had a bad attack of gout at the time and couldn't make it to most of the meetings, though he made significant contributions through a draft sent to him by Thomas Jefferson. Another signatory to the Declaration of Independence was John Hancock, a man who critics claimed used his gout as an excuse to hide away when things got difficult to avoid denting his popularity. A less popular figure, at least on the western side of the Atlantic, was Benedict Arnold. Arnold was a distinguished major general in the American Continental Army until he defected to the British and became one of the most notorious traitors in American history. It has been speculated that the constant pain in his gout-riven leg, not to mention the two bullet wounds he got in the same leg, drove him into the arms of the British.

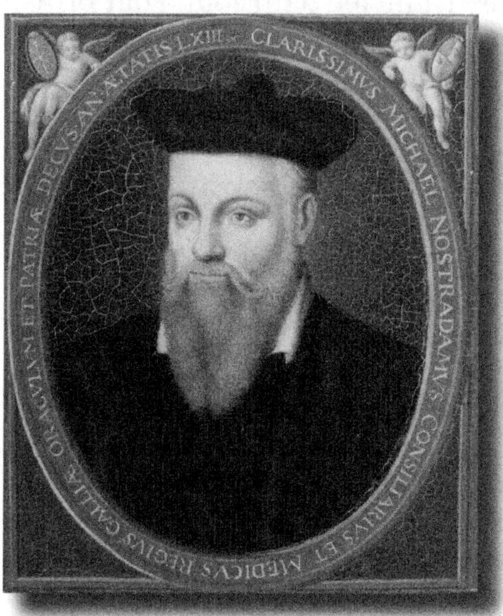

Figure 34: The French astrologer Nostradamus, famous for his book of prophecies, lost his life to gout.

Long before Franklin and Hancock, Christopher Columbus had had his own battles with gout – though some historians have suggested he may have actually had a reactive arthritis brought on either by food poisoning on his long voyages, or by a sexually transmitted infection. Another seafarer and adventurer, the hugely influential botanist Joseph Banks, who took part in Captain Cook's first great voyage and brought home 30,000 plant specimens from that and subsequent trips around the world, also had gout. He suffered from it every winter, eventually leading to him becoming wheelchair-bound.

Let us finish with the French astrologer Nostradamus, famous for his book of prophecies, who suffered from gout and arthritis much of his adult life and is said to have died from complications of his gout. I wonder if he saw that coming.

Chapter 43

Gout in culture

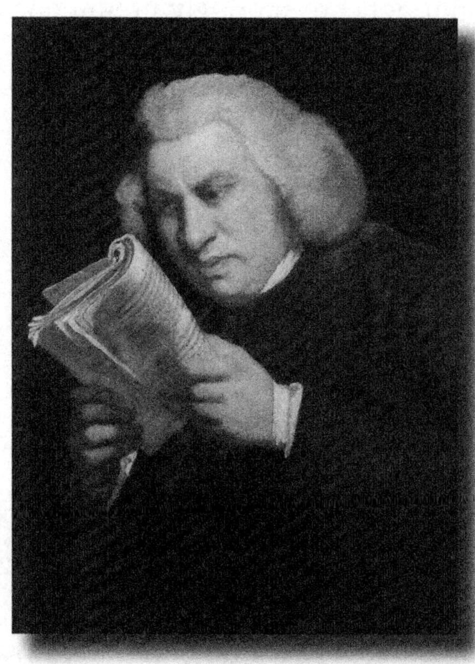

Figure 35: Samuel Johnson, creator of one of the first English dictionaries, spent the last few years of his life bed-ridden from gout.

A number of authors have lived with gout. Samuel Johnson, a British writer famous for writing a revolutionary new dictionary, suffered greatly from gout and was bed-ridden for the last few years of his life. The poet John Milton, author of Paradise Lost, is thought to have died of gout, and it left writer Henry Fielding on crutches. Joseph Conrad, author of Heart of Darkness (on which the film Apocalypse Now is based) and Lord Jim, was hospitalised for several months with gout. In Conrad's case, it affected his arm, making writing difficult - no small challenge for a writer. The poet Dylan Thomas also battled gout, as did Wilkie Collins, author of The Woman in White and Moonstone, considered the first modern English detective novel. He later became addicted to the opium he took to control the gout pain.

Gout makes an appearance in a few literary works too. In Charles Dickens's Great Expectations Clara Barley, a friend of Pip, lives with

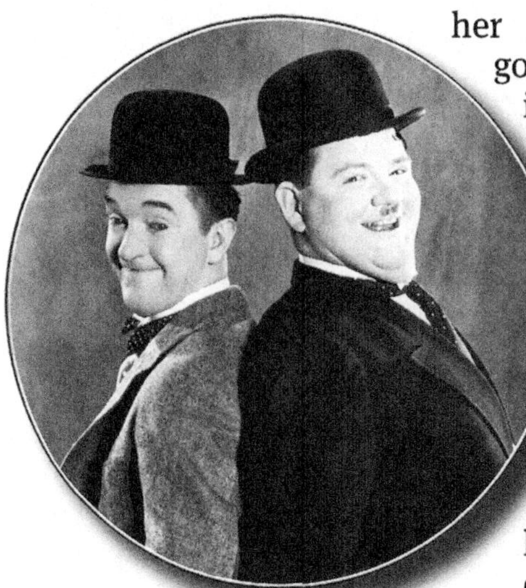

Figure 36: In Them Thar Hills, Ollie goes to the mountains to recover from gout, while Stan tags along to cause chaos.

her gout-ridden father, who treats his gout with "an abundance of rum", and in Jane Austen's Northanger Abbey, Mr Allen goes to Bath to be treated for his gout. At the time, Bath had recently grown in popularity after its Roman-era baths were re-opened for the treatment of gout. In more contemporary work, in Stephen King's novella Fair Extension, one of the protagonists, Tom Goodhugh, develops gout and psoriasis and in his suffering likens himself to Job, whilst in Game of Thrones, Doran Martell, the ruler of Dorne, battles gout as well as his neighbours.

Gout appears sparingly in film and TV too. In Caught in the Rain, Charlie Chaplin twice falls over the leg of a man with gout, whilst in Them, Thar Hills, Stan Laurel and Oliver Hardy travel to the mountains for Ollie to recover from his gout. More recently, in The Big Bang Theory, Mrs Wolowitz is occasionally bed-ridden with flare-ups of her gout, and in the British sitcom Keeping Up Appearances, Hyacinth is horrified to find that her husband Richard has come down with athlete's foot, something she considers frightfully lower class, so she insists he tells everyone it's gout, brought on by 'an excess of good living.' Gout features too in episodes of the American animated sitcom Central Park and in Dr Quinn, Medicine Woman. Olivia Colman won Best Actress awards at the Academy Awards, the Golden Globes and the BAFTAs for her portrayal of Queen Ann, sick with gout, in the 2018 film The Favourite.

Those making the films can be affected too. Actor Jared Leto had to gain 60 pounds for his role as Mark David Chapman, killer of John Lennon, in the film Chapter 27. As a

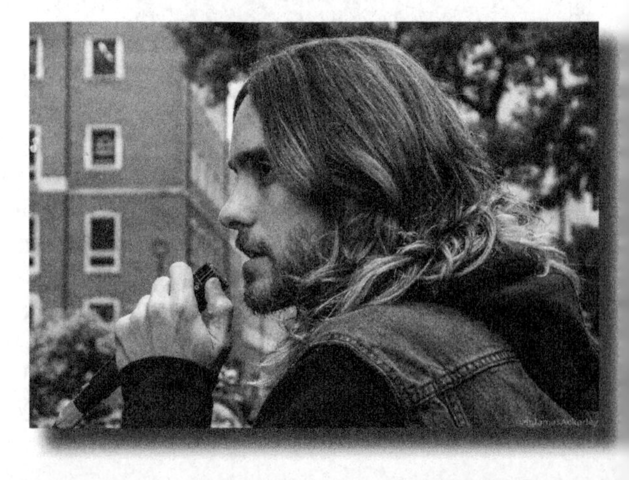

Figure 37: After putting on 60 lb for a film role, actor Jared Leto ended up in a wheelchair because of gout in his foot.

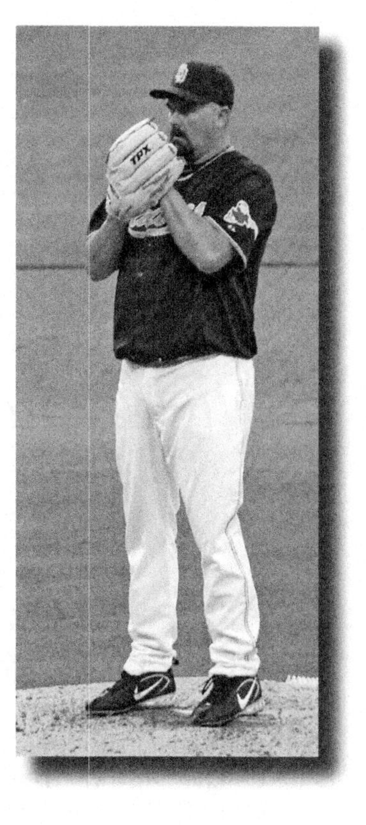

Figure 38: New York Yankees pitcher David Wells has talked openly about his challenges with gout.

result, he developed gout in his foot and, for a while, had to use a wheelchair. Oliver Reed's gout was no doubt made worse by his excess weight and drinking, and English comedian Mel Smith took an overdose of ibuprofen in an attempt to control the pain of his gout. Partly as a result of this, he was forced to sell his television production company Talkback Productions.

Despite being super fit, athletes are not immune from gout. David Wells, a pitcher for the New York Yankees and Toronto Blue Jays, has had to deal with gout for most of his career. NBA basketball player Maurice Cheeks developed gout at 46, and Australian footballer Harry Kewell was diagnosed with gout during the 2006 World Cup in Germany. American wrestler "Crusher" Jerry Blackwell suffered multiple complications associated with his weight, including gout and diabetes.

So, take heart. If your gout sometimes gets you down, just remember that you're in good company.

Chapter 44

Review your understanding

You will get the most effective medical care when you can have informed discussions with your doctor and other healthcare workers and make joint decisions about your treatment. You need a good understanding of the disease and its treatment to do that. The whole purpose of The Gout Handbook is to give you this understanding.

In this section, we provide you with eight case histories of patients who visited their doctors with various symptoms and complaints. Here is your chance to play the doctor's part, make a diagnosis, and decide what to do next. Each case is followed by some questions. Answers and explanations are provided, with references to the chapters covering the information in more detail.

Following the case histories is a quiz. Use the questions to test your understanding and refresh your memory.

Finally, there are a few crossword and wordfinder puzzles to help you remember the key words and concepts you should know.

We hope that revisiting the things you've read about in different ways will reinforce what you have learned and prepare you to have empowered conversations with your doctor.

Chapter 45

Case stories

Your turn to be the doctor

Case one: A rude awakening

George Dixon was woken in the early hours of the morning by a throbbing pain in his left big toe. When he examined his toe, it was warm and pink around the first joint and painful when he moved it. Unable to get back to sleep, he limped downstairs and made himself a cup of tea.

Over the morning, the pain got worse and worse. By lunchtime, the joint was clearly swollen and now a deep red and was agonisingly painful when he tried to walk. He could not face any lunch, and he was starting to feel hot and sweaty.

He couldn't understand what was going on. The pain in his big toe reminded him of how his hand had felt a couple of years ago when he'd accidentally slammed it in the car door, yet he hadn't injured it.

By four in the afternoon, he couldn't stand the pain any longer. His doctor couldn't see him until the next day, so he went to his local hospital's emergency department

a. What is the most likely diagnosis?

b. What other serious condition needs to be ruled out to avoid joint damage?

c. What is the most critical test needed to make a firm diagnosis?

d. What immediate treatment should George be given?

Case one: A rude awakening - Answers

a. The most likely diagnosis is gout. George has all the typical features: the rapid onset of a hot, red, swollen and excruciatingly painful joint. He also has a fever and feels generally unwell. His affected joint, the big toe, is the most commonly affected joint. (See page 13).

b. Although gout is the most likely diagnosis, there are other possibilities, including pseudogout, a bacterial joint infection and palindromic rheumatism. Of these, a bacterial joint infection must be excluded quickly because, if left untreated, it can cause severe damage to the joint. (See page 15).

c. The only way to rule out a joint infection and look for and identify crystals in joint fluid to make a firm diagnosis is to take a fluid sample from the affected joint, look at it under a microscope, and culture it to see if bacteria are present. (See page 24).

d. The priority is to relieve George's pain. He should be treated with either a non-steroidal anti-inflammatory drug or colchicine. An injection of steroids into the joint can give rapid relief but usually isn't used for a first attack until a bacterial infection has been ruled out. (See page 30).

Case two: Breaking the cycle

Mabel Johnson had her first attack of gout two years ago in her big toe. Since then, she's had three more episodes, two more in her big toe and one in her ankle. Now she's back at her doctor with a flareup in her wrist. Her flareups are treated with non-steroidal anti-inflammatory drugs and settle within a few days. However, she wants to reduce the number of attacks as they're very painful, and she has to take up to a week off work each time.

a. What medication would help reduce the frequency of Mable's gout attacks? (There are several choices).

b. When should the new medication start?

Case two: Breaking the cycle - Answers

a. Mabel and her doctor have several choices to reduce the frequency of her gout attacks.

   i. Mabel could take a low dose of a non-steroidal anti-inflammatory drug every day. (See page 34).

   ii. She could take colchicine once or twice a day. (See page 34).

   iii. She could take a drug that blocks the production of urate, the chemical that forms crystals in the joints. The most commonly used drug is allopurinol. (See page 36).

   iv. She could take a drug that increases the amount of urine she gets rid of in the urine each day. (See page 37).

b. A maintenance dose of a non-steroidal anti-inflammatory drug should be started as soon as the current attack has settled. Drugs to which reduce the amount of urate in the body, such as allopurinol, should be started as soon as the doctor determines that it is needed. In the past doctors thought starting too early could cause an acute attack to last longer, but that is not the case. (See page 35).

Case three: Changing up the menu

Sanjay Mehta's wife, Geeta, has come along with him today for his doctor's visit. Sanjay has had gout for three years, and his attacks are pretty well controlled. He has had only one episode in the last 18 months.

Sanjay takes allopurinol 300 mg once a day to reduce the amount of urate in his body, but his blood test shows that his blood uric acid level seems to be stuck at 6.5 mg/dL (0.39 mmol/L). Sanjay and his doctor would like his blood level to be lower.

Sanjay's wife has heard that certain foods can increase the urate level in the body. She wants to know what changes she should make to her cooking to help Sanjay's gout.

a. How would you advise Geeta? What foods should Sanjay avoid to help reduce his urate level?

b. Suppose the change in diet doesn't reduce Sanjay's uric acid levels enough. What else can Sanjay and his doctor do to reduce it further?

c. What blood level of uric acid should Sanjay be aiming for?

Case three: Changing up the menu - Answers

a. Sanjay should be avoiding foods rich in purines as these chemicals get broken down to urate in the body, and it's urate crystals that cause the problems in gout. Purine-rich foods that Sanjay should avoid include some red meats, especially organ meat like liver and kidney, dried mushrooms and yeast products. A diet rich in fruits, vegetables, nuts and grains will help keep Sanjay's urate level down. Geeta can check a more detailed list of the purine content of foods, such as the one on page 85 of this Handbook, to help her plan Sanjay's diet.

b. Eating a low purine diet might lower Sanjay's blood uric acid level by about 1 mg/dL (0.06 mmol/L). If that's not enough, there are more things that Sanjay and his doctor can do to reduce it further.

   i. Firstly, if Sanjay is overweight, he should make serious efforts to get back to a healthy weight. People who are overweight produce more urate, so less weight means less urate.

   ii. Sanjay is taking 300 mg of allopurinol each day. Increasing the dose will likely reduce his uric acid further. The maximum dose is 800 mg daily, so there is plenty of room to increase Sanjay's dose.

   iii. If this still doesn't bring Sanjay's levels down enough, the doctor can prescribe other drugs to block urate production or increase the amount of urate Sanjay excretes each day in the urine (See page 37).

c. If Sanjay does not have tophi, his blood uric acid level should be kept at or below 6 mg/dL (0.36 mmol per litre). If he does have tophi, it should be kept at or below 5 mg/dL (0.30 mmol/ litre) (See page 36).

Case four: No standing still

Theo Pacala had several severe gout attacks a few years ago, but he's only had one attack in the last two years. On his drive to work this morning, he developed severe pain in his left loin extending across his abdomen. It seemed to have mostly settled down by the time he got to work, but within an hour, it was back. A workmate found him pacing up and down the corridor, clearly in pain and looking grey. When Theo went to the bathroom, he noticed that his urine had a distinct pink tinge. Theo called the doctor for an urgent appointment.

a. What is the most likely cause of Theo's pain?

b. How will the doctor confirm the diagnosis?

c. What treatment does Theo need?

d. What can Theo do to prevent another episode like this?

Case four: No standing still - Answers

a. Theo's pain is most likely due to a kidney stone that has got stuck in the ureter between his kidney and bladder (See page 68).

b. The most effective way to confirm a diagnosis of kidney stones is with a spiral/helical CT scan. An ultrasound scan can also be used. An x-ray of the abdomen may show a kidney stone, but it is less useful for urate kidney stones which may be invisible to x-rays (See page 68).

c. The first priority is to control Theo's pain. This is usually first achieved with an injection of a powerful painkiller, followed by oral painkillers.
Most people will pass the stone on their own within 6 to 8 weeks. Sometimes the doctor will prescribe medication to relax the ureter, to make it easier to pass the stone, and occasionally will prescribe medication to make the urine more alkaline, which helps dissolve urate stones. If the stone does not pass, it can be broken up into smaller pieces using powerful ultrasound shock waves or removed using an instrument inserted via the bladder (See page 71).

d. Reducing the amount of urate in Theo's body will reduce the risk of further stones. This can be done by lowering production with a drug like allopurinol. (Drugs that increase urate excretion can make kidney stones worse by increasing the amount of urate in the urine.) He should also avoid purine-rich foods that get broken down to urate in the body and drink at least six pints/three litres of fluid a day to reduce crystal formation in the urine.

Case five: Gout behaving rashly

Ken Chan had an attack of gout about six months ago. A blood test showed that his uric acid level was high at 9 mg/dl /0.54 mmol/L, so two weeks ago, Ken's doctor prescribed him allopurinol to reduce the amount of urate he produces and hence to lower the blood level.

A couple of days ago, Ken developed a red, itchy rash on his upper chest, neck and face, which has been steadily getting worse.

a. What is the most likely cause of Ken's rash?

b. What should Ken do?

Case five: Gout behaving rashly - Answers

a. Ken's rash is most likely to be an uncommon but potentially serious reaction to allopurinol (See page 36)

b. Ken should contact his doctor immediately and stop taking the allopurinol until a doctor has seen him. If the rash is due to allopurinol and Ken keeps taking it, it could become a much more severe reaction.

Case six: One lump or two?

Burt Goodman had his first attack of gout five years ago. He gets an attack about once a year, and they settle in a few days with non-steroidal anti-inflammatory medication. He doesn't consider this a major inconvenience, so he doesn't take any preventative medicine.

Recently Burt noticed a firm lump under the skin of his left elbow and then a pale yellow, firm nodule under the skin in his right ear lobe. They are not painful or causing any problems.

a. What do you think these nodules are?

b. Is treatment necessary?

Case six: One lump or two? - Answers

a. Burt's nodules are likely to be tophi. These are collections of urate crystals in the tissues. They tend to occur in the cooler parts of the body and can sometimes occur in joints (See page 43).

b. Treatment isn't essential if the tophi aren't bothering Burt. However, they may indicate high levels of urate in Burt's body. That increases his risk of more frequent gout attacks and also of getting kidney stones. Tophi can also occur in joints and may cause joint damage. Bert should talk to his doctor, who will probably do a blood test to measure Burt's uric acid level. They can then discuss the possibility of putting Burt on medication to reduce the urate level. In time this will lead to the disappearance of his tophi (page 43).

Case seven: More than a touch of heartburn

Stella Cambray had her second attack of gout a couple of weeks ago. She took high-dose non-steroidal anti-inflammatory drugs for a week to control the pain and swelling during the attack. She then continued with a lower dose to prevent another attack.

During the attack, she developed indigestion which has been getting worse and has started keeping her awake at night. Three days ago, she noticed that her stools had become very dark, almost black. Today she vomited, and her stomach contents looked like coffee grounds.

a. What do you think is the cause of Stella's indigestion, dark stools and 'coffee ground' vomiting?

b. What should Stella do?

Case seven: More than a touch of heartburn - Answers

a. The black colour of Stella's stools and 'coffee ground' vomiting are both due to the presence of blood that has been altered by the action of stomach acid. Non-steroidal anti-inflammatory drugs can sometimes irritate the stomach lining. As an uncommon but serious side-effect, this can lead to ulcers and/or bleeding (See page 86).

b. Bleeding into the gastrointestinal tract should be considered an emergency. Stella should contact her doctor immediately or go to the local hospital emergency department. It is most likely that if she contacts her doctor, she will be sent to the hospital so the site and cause of bleeding can be determined (See page 86)

Case eight: A suddenly painful knee

Since around the time she retired, Margaret Hoskins has been troubled by aching pains in several toes, her left wrist, and her right knee.

Yesterday her right knee became a lot more painful over the course of the morning. She can still bend her knee and walk on it, but it's a lot more painful than usual. Apart from the pain in her knee, Margaret feels fine.

a. What might be the cause of Margaret's painful knee?

b. How will Margaret's doctor make a diagnosis?

c. What treatment should Margaret receive?

Case eight: A suddenly painful knee - Answers

a. Several different conditions could be the cause of Margaret's painful knee. Gout is certainly a possibility though her knee isn't as painful as you might expect with gout. That, and the fact that it's her knee that's affected, make pseudogout a possibility. As always with a suddenly painful joint, an infection needs to be considered. An injury is another possible cause; there is no suggestion of that here. There are several other possibilities too, so some investigations will be required to make a firm diagnosis (See page 106).

b. To investigate the possibility of gout, pseudogout, or a joint infection, some fluid should be taken from the knee and examined under the microscope. The fluid should also be cultured to see if any bacteria are present. Margaret has had an aching knee for a while, so x-rays may be helpful to see if there are signs of wear and tear or other damage. In this case, rod-shaped crystals of CPPD were seen in the joint fluid, making a diagnosis of pseudogout (See page 108).

c. Pseudogout is usually treated with non-steroidal anti-inflammatory drugs. Colchicine may be used as an alternative. (See page 110).

Chapter 46

Quiz

1. Gout is caused by crystals of which chemical in the joints or other tissues?

    a. Sodium chloride
    b. Allopurinol
    c. Urate
    d. Calcium oxalate
    e. Glucose

2. Which of the following is not a symptom of gout?

    a. A swollen joint
    b. Fever and chills
    c. Severe joint pain
    d. A rash
    e. A joint that's hot and red

3. Which of these groups are most likely to get gout?

    a. Women
    b. People who are overweight
    c. Young people
    d. Sportsmen and women
    e. People who have had previous joint surgery

4. Which of these foods is not known to increase blood uric acid levels?

    a. Beer
    b. Meat gravy and broths
    c. Sardines and mussels
    d. Yeast extract
    e. Coffee

5. Gout attacks only occur in the big toe.

    a. True
    b. False

6. Tophi are lumps or nodules that can occur in various tissues due to an accumulation of urate crystals.

    a. True
    b. False

7. Which of these is not a common site for tophi?

    a. Nose
    b. Fingers
    c. Achilles tendon
    d. Ear lobes
    e. Joints

8. Conditions that may cause similar symptoms to gout include:

    a. A joint infection
    b. Palindromic rheumatism
    c. Lyme Disease
    d. Psoriasis
    e. All of the above

9. Examination of joint fluid from an affected joint is the only way to tell the difference with certainty between gout, pseudogout and a joint infection.

    a. True
    b. False

10. Which of the following is true?

    a. Someone with a high blood uric acid level will eventually develop gout.
    b. If someone had a painful joint but a normal blood uric acid level, the cause cannot be gout.
    c. The blood uric acid does not help guide gout treatment.
    d. None of the above.

11. Measurement of the amount of urate passed in the urine over 24 hours can help determine if a person's high uric levels are due to producing too much urate or not excreting enough in the urine

    a. True
    b. False

12. Which of the following medicines can be used to treat a gout attack?

    a. Non-steroidal anti-inflammatory drugs
    b. Colchicine
    c. Steroids
    d. Anakinra
    e. All of the above

13. Which of the following does not help treat an attack of gout?

    a. Resting the joint
    b. Splinting the joint
    c. Applying hot towels to the joint
    d. Taking painkillers
    e. Putting an ice pack on the joint

14. Which of the following is not an effective way to reduce the amount of urate in the body?

    a. Avoiding foods that are broken down to urate in the body.
    b. Taking medicines that block the production of urate.
    c. Taking medicines that increase the excretion of your rate in the urine.
    d. Taking non-steroidal anti-inflammatory drugs.
    e. Getting down to a healthy weight, if overweight.

15. Which of these medicines can occasionally have side effects that include indigestion, gastrointestinal bleeding, impairment of kidney function and an increased risk of a heart attack?

    a. Allopurinol
    b. Colchicine
    c. Febuxostat
    d. Paracetamol/acetaminophen
    e. Non-steroidal anti-inflammatory drugs

16. The dose of allopurinol used to reduce the body's uric level is 300 mg once-a-day

    a. True
    b. False

17. For someone with tophi on medication to reduce the level of urate in the body, what is the ideal blood uric acid level to aim for?

    a. Greater than 8mg/dL (0.48 mmol/L)
    b. 7 – 8 mg/dL (0.42 – 0.48 mmol/L)
    c. 6-7 mg/dL (0.36 – 0.42 mmol/L)
    d. 5 – 6 mg/dL (0.30 – 0.36 mmol/L)
    e. 5 mg/dL (0.30 mmol/L) or less

18. Approximately what proportion of people with gout develop kidney stones?

    a. Almost all
    b. 1 in 5
    c. 1 in 50
    d. 1 in 100
    e. None

19. Which of the following is not a symptom of kidney stones?

    a. Severe pain in the loin
    b. Feeling breathless
    c. Pink or red urine
    d. Not being able to stay still
    e. Vomiting

20. Most people with kidney stones need to have the stone broken into pieces with high power ultrasound waves or removed through an instrument.

    a. True
    b. False

21. Treatment with a drug to reduce the amount of urate in the body (allopurinol, for example) should not be started until an attack of gout has completely resolved.

    a. True
    b. False

22. Gout and pseudogout are easy to tell apart based on their symptoms

    a. True
    b. False

23. Which of the following is a reason to contact your doctor immediately:

    a. A rash while taking allopurinol
    b. Severe indigestion, vomiting blood or 'coffee grounds', or passing black stools
    c. Severe loin pain, passing urine frequently, and/or pink or red urine
    d. A gout attack that feels quite different from previous episodes or which is taking longer than usual to settle
    e. All of the above

24. Which of the following statements is true:

    a. Gout is more common in women
    b. Pseudogout mainly affects young people
    c. Gout affects primarily young people
    d. Pseudogout attacks men and women equally
    e. Gout and pseudogout are both caused by the same type of crystal

25. Colchicine taken every day can reduce the frequency of attacks of both gout and pseudogout

    a. True
    b. False

Quiz - Answers

1. c. Urate

   Gout is caused by crystals of monosodium urate, or urate for short. (See page 4)

2. d. A rash

   A rash is not a feature of gout. A rash may be a side effect of allopurinol. It may progress to a more severe reaction if allopurinol is continued. The other symptoms are features of gout. (See page 13)

3. c. People who are overweight.

   The risk of gout increases in proportion to your body mass index (BMI). Essentially, the rounder you are, the more likely you are to get gout. You're also more likely to have recurrent attacks. (See page 11)

4. e. Coffee

   Drinking coffee lowers your blood uric acid levels. Drink away! (See page 85 and page 125)

5. b. False

   Although gout very commonly affects the first joint of the big toe, it can affect many other joints, including the instep, ankle, knee, wrist and elbow. Rarely the hip, pelvic, shoulder, collar bone and neck joints may be affected. (See page 13)

6. a. True

   Tophi are caused by urate crystals accumulating in the skin, joints and other tissues. (See page 43)

7. a. Nose

Tophi tend to occur in the cooler parts of the body, most likely because urate is less soluble at cooler temperatures. For some reason, the nose seems to be spared – thank goodness. (See page 43)

8. e. All of the above

Many conditions can give similar symptoms to gout. That's why it's so important to get a rock-solid diagnosis by examining fluid from an affected joint for urate crystals. (See page 15)

9. a. True

Many other conditions can mimic gout. The only way to be sure of the diagnosis is to examine fluid from an affected joint to look for urate crystals. Since you are likely to be embarking on life-long treatment, it is crucial to get the diagnosis correct. (See page 24)

10. d. None of the above

It is undoubtedly true that having a high uric acid level does make you more likely to develop gout and to have recurrent attacks once you have gout. However, many people have a high uric acid level but do not have gout, and others have gout attacks with a normal uric acid level. (See page 27)

Uric acid levels are very helpful in guiding treatment to lower the amount of urate in the body. The dose of medication is adjusted to bring the uric acid level into the target range. (See page 36)

11. a. True

Most people with gout have high urate levels because they do not excrete enough urate in the urine. For some, the problem is producing too much. The way to tell the difference is to measure the amount of urate passed in the urine in 24 hours. (See page 27)

12. e. All of the above

    All of these medicines can be used to treat an acute attack of gout. (See page 30)

13. c. Applying hot towels to the joint

    Most people find that applying an ice pack to a joint affected by a gout attack is soothing. On the contrary, very few people find that applying heat to the joint helps. This difference is so marked that it has even been suggested as a way of telling the difference between gout and other conditions that can cause inflamed joints. (See page 34)

14. d. Non-steroidal anti-inflammatory drugs

    Non-steroidal anti-inflammatory drugs can effectively prevent gout attacks, but they do this through their anti-inflammatory effect, not by reducing the amount of urate in the body. The other measures do lessen the body's urate load. (See page 36)

15. e. Non-steroidal anti-inflammatory drugs

    Although non-steroidal anti-inflammatory drugs are incredibly useful medicines, they can cause serious problems if not used correctly and monitored appropriately. The risk of side effects is significantly increased in older adults. (See page 30)

16. b. False

    For many doctors, 300 mg is a standard dose of allopurinol, but there is no such thing as a standard dose – it needs to be adjusted to fit the patient's needs. The correct dose of allopurinol is the one that brings your blood uric acid level into the target range. The dose can be increased to a maximum of 800 mg per day. Too many people are on too low of a dose, putting them at risk of attacks that could have been avoided and long term complications of gout such as kidney stones and joint damage. (See page 36 and page 45).

17. e. 5 mg/dL (0.30 mmol/L) or less

The target blood uric acid levels are 5 mg/dL (0.30 mmol/L) or less if you have tophi and 6 mg/dL (0.36 mmol/L) or less if you do not have tophi. The reason for the lower level if you have tophi is that this allows the urate crystals in the tophi to dissolve and be removed so that the tophi get smaller and eventually disappear. (See page 35)

18. b. 1 in 5

Twenty per cent, that is one in five, people with gout will develop kidney stones. Kidney stones occur because urate is poorly soluble and so forms crystals in the urine. These crystals slowly enlarge over time as more urate forms around them. This is why it's essential to keep well hydrated if you have gout. Higher volumes of water passing through the kidneys can keep more urate dissolved, thus reducing the risk of crystals forming. (See page 68).

19. b. Feeling breathless

Feeling breathless is not a symptom of kidney stones. Someone with a kidney stone stuck in the ureter typically has excruciating pain causing them to stay constantly on the move, nausea and vomiting. They may look ashen and may pass blood-stained urine. (See page 68).

20. b. False

Most people will pass the stone on their own, perhaps with the help of a drug that relaxes the ureter, making it easier for the stone to pass through. Only a minority will need the stone to be broken up by high power ultrasound waves or removed surgically. (See page 71)

21. b. False

For a long time, it was believed that starting a drug to reduce urate levels during an acute gout attack would prolong the gout attack. Hence, the medicine should not be started until a few weeks or months after an attack. Many doctors still believe this. However, studies have shown that starting urate-lowering medication early does not prolong an attack, so it should be started as soon as it has been shown to be needed. (See page 35).

22. b. False

The symptoms of gout and pseudogout can be identical. This is one of the reasons why it is critical to get a firm diagnosis by examining fluid from an affected joint. (See page 106)

23. e. All of the above

A rash caused by allopurinol can progress to a more severe reaction if the allopurinol is not stopped. Severe indigestion, vomiting blood or 'coffee grounds' or passing black stools is likely due to stomach inflammation or a stomach ulcer and can be caused by non-steroidal anti-inflammatory drugs. Severe loin pain and passing pink or red urine are likely signs of either kidney stones or a kidney infection. One in five people with gout develops kidney stones. If a gout attack feels quite different from previous attacks, it may not be gout. It may be something that needs urgent attention, like a joint infection. Each of these scenarios requires a quick diagnosis and appropriate treatment, hence the need to see a doctor straight away. (See page 86).

24. d. Pseudogout affects men and women equally.

Unlike gout, which is three times more common in men, pseudogout is an equal opportunities disease, affecting men and women equally. (See page 104).

25. a. True

Colchicine can be effective at preventing attacks of both gout and pseudogout. (See page 32 and page 111).

Chapter 47

Puzzles

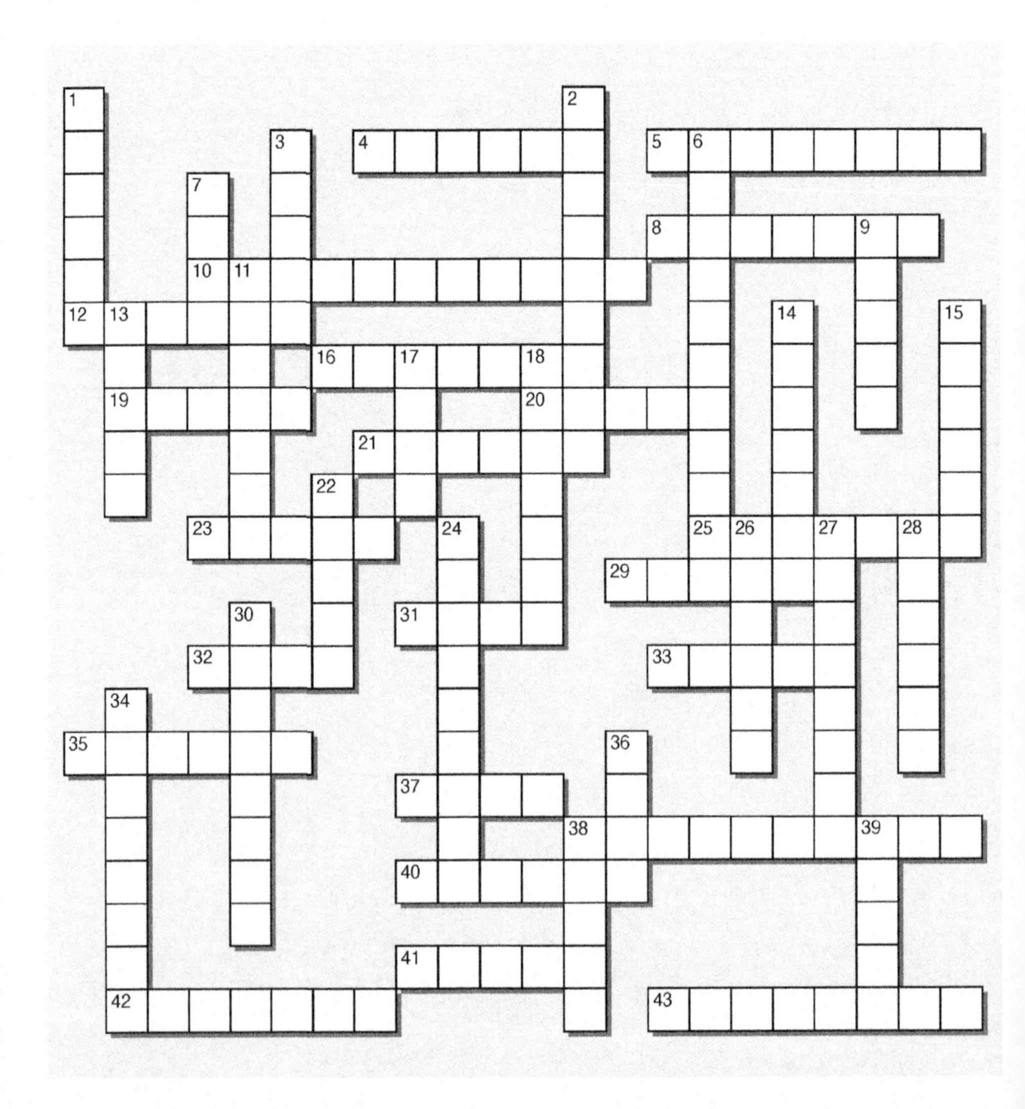

Across

4. The parts of the body affected by gout and pseudogout.

5. One of the typical sites for tophi.

8. Another word commonly used to describe an acute gout attack.

10. This variety of rheumatism can perfectly mimic gout.

12. Your doctor should use one of these to get a sample of joint fluid to look for crystals and make a cast-iron diagnosis.

16. These chemicals in food get broken down to urate in the body.

19. Uric acid levels in this fluid are used to adjust the dose of allopurinol.

20. One of the foods on the 'avoid' list if you have gout.

21. The abbreviation for a family of medicines very commonly used to treat gout.

23. This should be taken from a joint and examined for crystals to confirm a diagnosis of gout or pseudogout.

25. One of the big risk factors for gout.

29. Using one of these to rest a joint can be very helpful in an acute gout attack.

31. Kidney stones are not always visible on one of these.

32. The disease caused when urate crystals form in joints and other tissues.

33. You should try to drink two to three litres of this each day to reduce the risk of kidney stones.

35. Colchicine is made from this flower.

37. The drink you have to wave bye-bye to if you have gout.

38. An alternative to allopurinol.

40. Drinking this popular beverage reduces your risk of further attacks.

41. Urate is removed from the body in this fluid.

42. NSAIDs can cause serious irritation or even ulcers in this part of the body.

43. Eating these several times a week may offer protection from gout attacks.

Down

1. Which famous English poet was not in Paradise with his painful foot?

2. This skin disease can also cause arthritis.

3. Gout doesn't just affect the big toe. It gets this joint too.

6. Name the drug most commonly used to reduce the amount of urate in the body?

7. Crystals of this chemical cause pseudogout.

9. Gout is due to crystals of this chemical in the joints and other tissues.

11. One of our favorite recreational substances, but doubly bad for us if we have gout.

13. Yet another joint that gout can affect.

14. In an acute gout attack, the affected joint often looks like this.

15. One in five people with gout gets stones in these.

17. If you develop one of these while taking allopurinol, you must see your doctor immediately.

18. This group of people are especially susceptible to drug side effects.

22. All too often, an attack of gout will start at this time of day.

24. This actor developed gout after piling on 60 lb for a film role.

26. The classic site for a gout attack.

27. These can be injected into an inflamed joint in gout and pseudogout.

28. The singular form of tophi.

30. Name the European 'discoverer' of the Americas who battled gout.

34. Gout and pseudogout are both caused by these forming in the joints.

36. The joint most often affected by pseudogout.

38. This can be a feature of both gout and pseudogout.

39. These collections of urate in the tissues cause nodules in the skin, joints and earlobes.

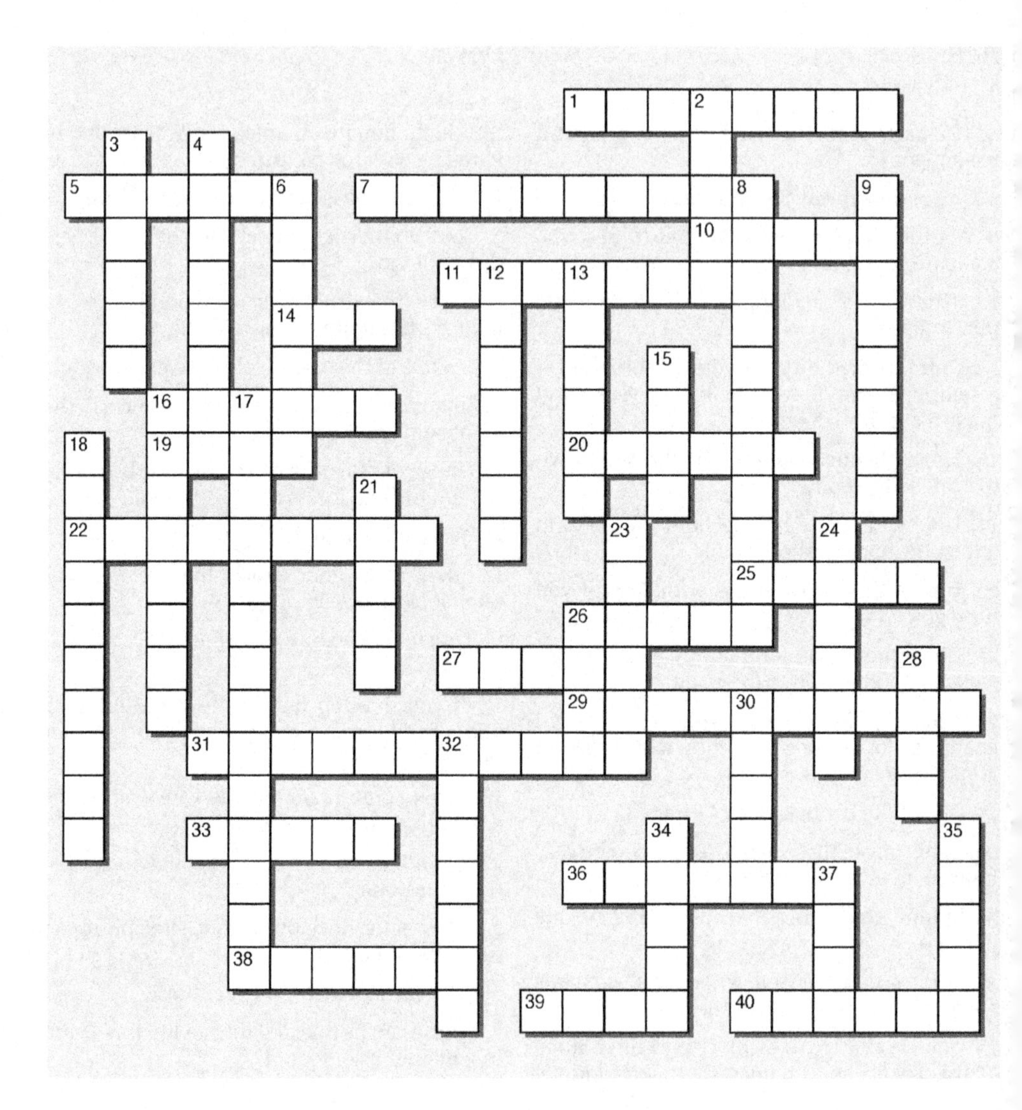

Across

1. In 1492 this explorer 'sailed the ocean blue' while doing battle with gout.

5. Gout can affect a variety of these.

7. This celebrated Mongol leader suffered greatly from gout.

10. Usually, these collections of urate in tissues will slowly dissolve and disappear if the blood uric acid level is kept low.

11. Nodules on these may be a sign of gout.

Down

2. In some people with gout, crystals of this chemical form tophi.

3. What you call tophi when there is only one.

4. A medicine given by injection to treat gout attacks if the usual medications are not working.

6. You should take NSAIDs with a full glass of water to ensure that they reach this.

14. The people who are most affected by gout.

16. The flower from which colchicine is made.

19. This can occur if you are taking allopurinol. You should talk to your doctor right away.

20. This family of drugs can be used to treat a gout attack and to prevent future attacks.

22. This sweet-smelling resin relieves osteoarthritis pain but hasn't been adequately tested for gout.

25. Eating food that makes this more alkaline can help remove urate from the body.

26. Perhaps 50% of our risk of getting gout comes from these.

27. In someone with kidney stones, this can sometimes be seen in the urine.

29. This can be an excellent way to look for kidney stones.

31. In which 2019 award-winning film about Queen Anne and her maidservants did gout play a starring role?

33. The favorite time for a gout attack to begin.

36. In gout, these happen more often in spring than any other season.

38. You can improvise one of these for the big toe by tying it loosely to the next toe.

39. A few pints of this at the pub can really increase your chances of a gout attack.

40. What a joint can feel like during an acute attack.

8. Which famous French astrologer of the 1500s suffered terribly from gout?

9. People who eat these have less gout attacks.

12. We may love this, but it makes the liver produce more urate, and stops the kidney getting rid of urate. Bad news all round.

13. This citrus fruit is often recommended for gout, but there's no solid evidence that it works.

15. In someone with gout, these can show holes in the bones that look as though they have been chewed by a rat.

16. Because uric acid is not very soluble, it readily forms these in the kidneys and other tissues.

17. This form of arthritis, which is more common in older adults, sometimes causes lumps on the fingers that can look like tophi.

18. You should have regular blood tests to monitor your liver if you take this medicine to block urate production.

21. The drug febuxostat, used to block urate production, can occasionally cause toxicity to this organ.

23. Urate crystals are this shape when seen under the microscope.

24. Pseudogout can affect this joint, making it easy to confuse it with gout.

26. This condition has been described as one of the worst treated chronic diseases.

28. Pseudogout often effects this joint.

30. One of the joints that can be affected by gout.

32. This makes gout more likely, and flare-ups more common.

34. Drinking two or three litres a day of this helps flush urate out of the body.

35. This, along with a sore throat and bleeding, can be a sign of bone marrow suppression, a serious but rare complication of some gout medicines.

37. This might wake you up at night in an acute attack.

C F P S E U D O G O U T T A T S O X U B E F
J C N W R A P U R I N E S U S E B O L R A E
B D V W O D N U O S A R T L U B S U C O R C
O K T Q S C M V F I T O P H U S N N L X E D
S U N A E X U P S O R I A S I S T I R Y A X
W B U P L Q S Y J D I C A C I R U A G V J O
E L B R U C N S S O C E E A G O D P I H B L
L A P W A S O I F O I L T I A E E D Y E T T
L I L A I T U H F L K N T I L R W E S A O C
I K K J L D E Z O N A E T D R E N I F P R B
A H F R A I I D A L N R E S L O T I H F L X
V A O L E D N C B D I E E L D Y V I K O O T
T N C A U V G D E F N T S U E H J A O A H C
F U I V K I I R R N E B H E P Q C D F H N C
K E R I W T D L F O E T G O S Q M A J E O A
Y I V M G E N E S L M B I N T E R O M D H O
L R R E E S D I Y E L I O S N R I K T O X T
R Z E X R R N E L V U W C R D W I R F Z T K
E I E T G H I O W P V G T R P I S P R R N S
D Y B I A K S C M L S U M K T Z A P S E C T
L K Z G S W Y A P E O X U R I N E S E Y H E
E N O E M B U D R G L P O M G T I L N L T C

ALCOHOL
ANAKINRA
ANKLE
BEER
BLOOD
BOSWELLIA
CHERRIES
COFFEE
CROCUS
DAVID WELLS
EARLOBES
ELDERLY
FEBUXOSTAT
FEVER
FLARE-UP
FLUID
GENES
GOUT
JOINTS
KNEE
KUBLAI KHAN
LEMONS
LITHOTRIPSY
LIVER
MEN
NEEDLE
NIGHT
NSAIDS
OBESITY
PAIN
PALINDROMIC
PROBENECID
PSEUDOGOUT
PSORIASIS
PURINES
RASH
SPLINT
STOMACH
TENDER
THE FAVORITE
TOPHI
TOPHUS
TURMERIC
ULTRASOUND
URATE
URIC ACID
URINE
WATER
X-RAY

```
N E E D L E D U R D I C A C I R U T O A R G
A S P A L I N D R O M I C I A I H P O T E T
E L L A T U O G O D U E S P N G X N G N O Q
V L C L Q Y M N Q R S N V O K M Q N E P W S
Z G D O E E F L U I D I W S L Q W S H T T U
I B F E H W O C V R Q A P T E S G U H E O L
H V C B R O D T V P F P V E E D S G R S I Z
T E E X I L L I G E E F F O C O I O U V Q F
N E D M O W Y I V I I T C A J N I C E B E W
M O N S A I D S U A B S B R O D O R F V Q L
P E S D R K L O U F D P P T S R G I E W I R
U O A T E T L Y V R R Y R H C E F R A T K Y
R T T R R R I O F Q I B U R N K S T H D N A
A N D G L A C K N I X N Z I A P E O N U H R
T A E C J O D S U I S Z E T L R T H O A S X
E R S P I H B A E R R H F I C R C P I H L R
S N I U Y R C E M I Q U N S I Z N R T E A C
T I R E E E E A S U R T P P N I G D C E T V
N K A R R V N M M V S R S O H R O L E N S W
I A L A O E N D R O D Y E A L O U B F K Y H
O N O L Y E E R I U T F B H L L T R N G R X
J A P F M M V B F K T S M B C D A J I O C M
```

ALCOHOL
ALLOPURINOL
ANAKINRA
ANKLE
BEER
BIGTOE
BLOOD
CHERRIES
COFFEE
CROCUS
CRYSTALS
DAVID WELLS
EARLOBES
ELDERLY
FEVER
FLAREUP
FLUID
GENES
GOUT
INFECTION
JOINTS
KIDNEY
KNEE
LITHOTRIPSY
LIVER
MEN
NEEDLE
NIGHT
NOSTRADAMUS
NSAIDS
OILY FISH
OSTEOARTHRITIS
PAIN
PALINDROMIC
POLARISED
PSEUDOGOUT
SPLINT
STEROIDS
STOMACH
TENDER
TOPHI
TOPHUS
TURMERIC
URATE
URIC ACID
URINE
WATER
XRAY

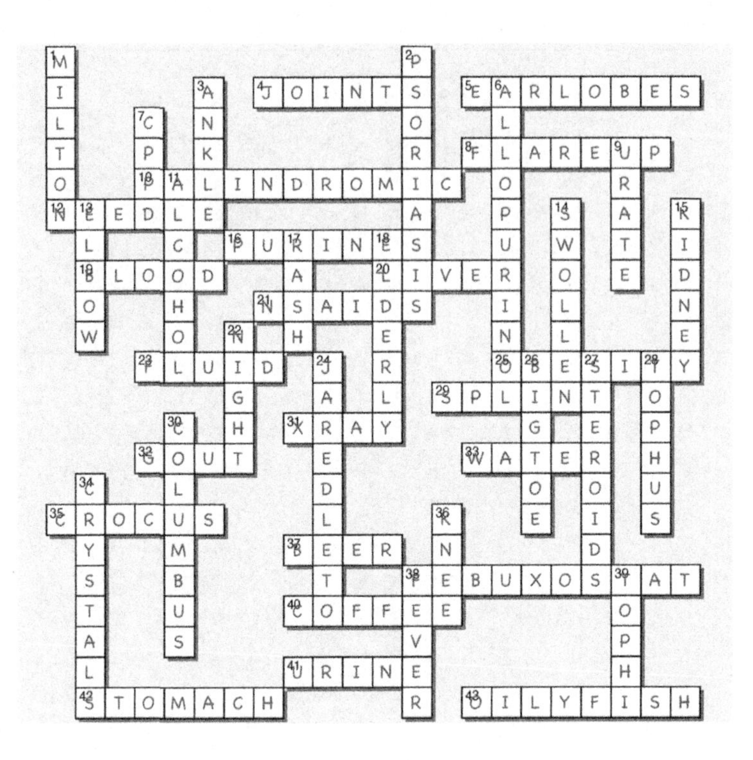

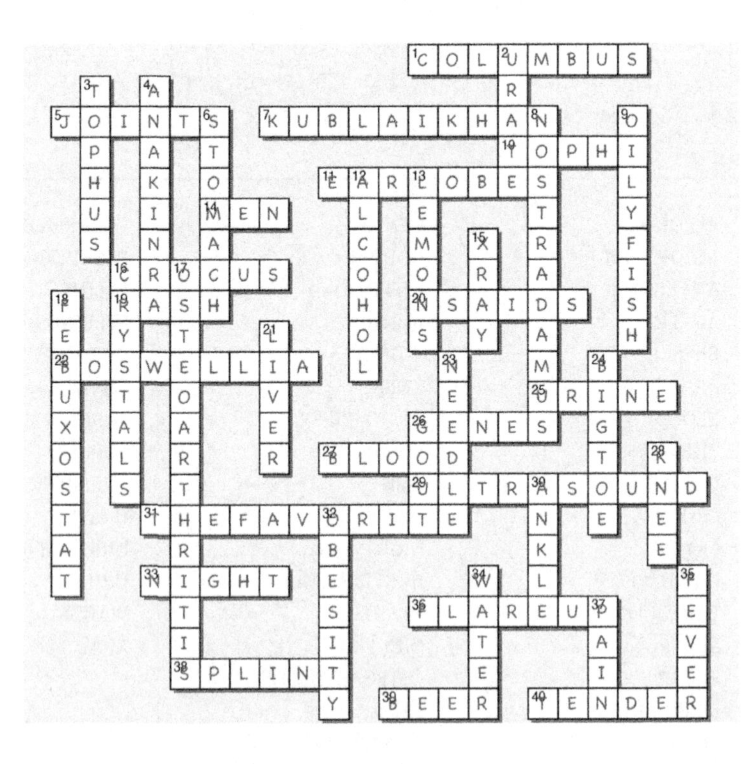

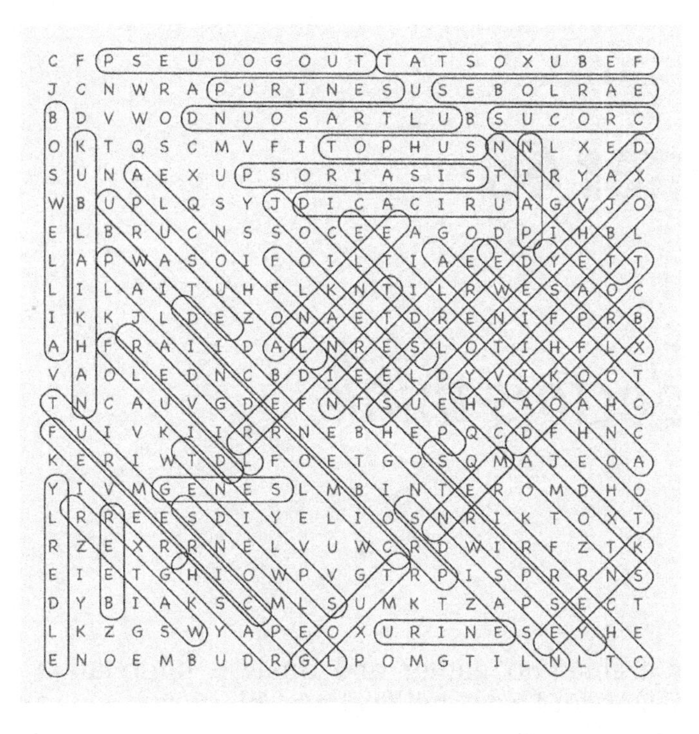

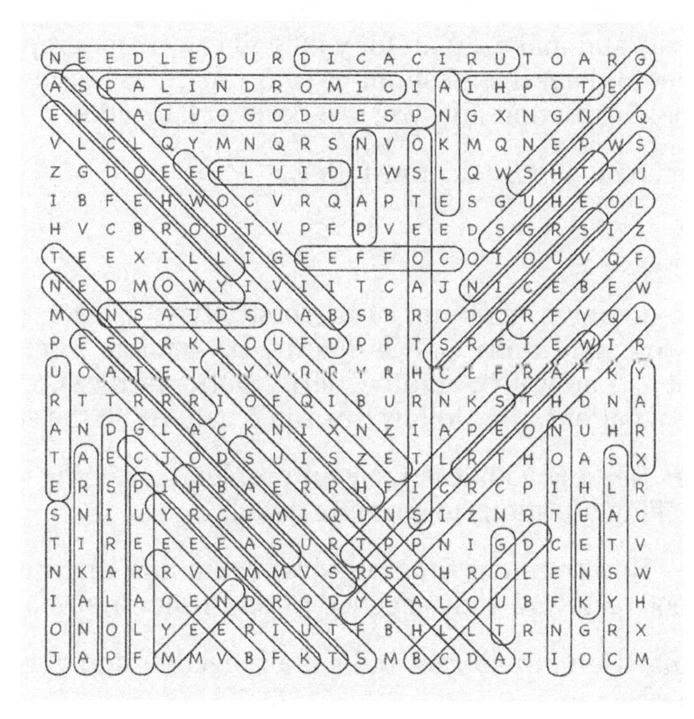

Chapter 48

How doctors think

Doctors are trained to gather and analyse information from their patients in a standard way – all doctors. This means you can learn how doctors think. If you understand how doctors think through a health issue, process and piece together all the information in order to arrive at a diagnosis and make a plan for you, you can better prepare for your appointment and get the most out of your time. You'll know what your doctor is looking for and how you can best work together.

Let's review the pattern doctors follow.

SOAP

SOAP is an acronym made up of the first letters of each stage of the medical assessment process. SOAP is the US version. Doctors in other countries may know it by another term, but regardless, every time a doctor sees a patient, they follow this same pattern, in the same order:

Subjective: Hearing you describe your problem. Listening to your story and then asking questions to get more detail.

Objective: This comprises the physical exam and any investigations such as blood tests and x-rays needed to get further information.

Assessment: Here, the doctor pulls it all together and gives it a name - the diagnosis.

Plan: The "to do" list for treating and resolving your health issues.

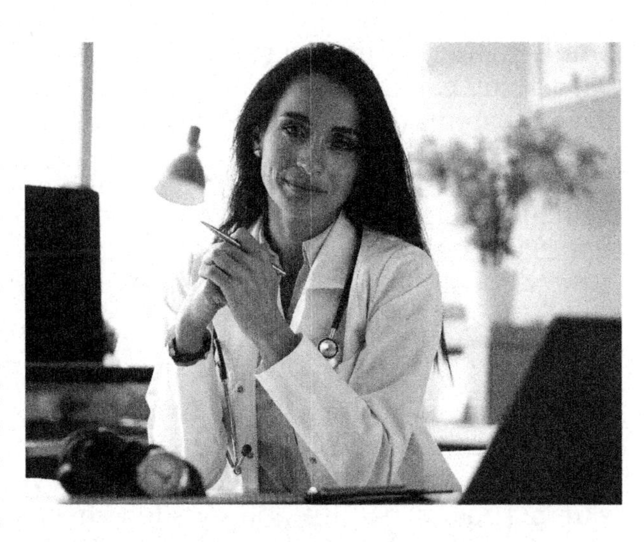

Notice this makes the acronym "SOAP". Let's take a closer look at each step, so you'll know what to expect and how to communicate effectively.

Subjective: Here, the doctor wants to learn more about you and your concerns. The first question asked will be about why you are in the clinic or hospital today. Then comes further questioning to get more detail. This is the critical stage of your appointment. Most seasoned doctors will have a fair idea of what's wrong within minutes of this conversation starting. Each symptom is weighed and considered. In his mind, something called a differential diagnosis is being formed, essentially a list of "what could this be?" As you speak, this differential diagnosis takes shape, with some items on the list being eliminated while others are added. The entire list gets put into priority of "most likely" to "least likely." This list is fine-tuned with every question you answer. You must be honest, forthcoming, and complete in the information you provide.

Around this time, your doctor will gather secondary information to help him complete your story. He may ask about:

Past medical history: Are you diabetic? Do you have high blood pressure? Do you suffer from anxiety or depression? Are there any other medical issues you've been dealing with? Have you ever been hospitalized, and if so, why? Your current health issue may be related to a past or ongoing condition. For example, someone with high blood pressure is at a higher risk for strokes and heart attacks.

Past surgical history: Similarly, this provides the doctor with clues that may explain what you're experiencing. For example, you may have had surgery on your abdomen years ago. Further down the road, this may lead to a hernia, resulting in abdominal pain or discomfort.

Medications: Most medicines have side effects. Your doctor might recognize an explanation or a contributing factor to your illness. Your doctor will want to know what you're taking, not just prescribed medications but also over-the-counter drugs and any supplements or herbal remedies. He'll ask you too about any allergies to medicines.

Family history: Since many medical issues are inherited, your doctor will ask you about medical conditions in your family. What health issues do your parents deal with? If they are no longer living, how did they die?

Social history: Knowing your occupation, where you live, home dynamics and how you spend your day adds another layer of information that might be helpful. Certain jobs or living conditions can make you more susceptible to certain diseases and offer explanations for your health issues.

At this point, in many clinical encounters, your doctor will do a "systems review." He'll be asking you open-ended questions about different parts of your body (or "systems") to jog your memory about anything you've not mentioned. So, even if you go to the doctor because your big toe is painful and swollen, he'll ask questions about your breathing, digestion, and nervous system. He is turning over every rock to complete the picture. Countless times, in this head-to-toe review, a patient will respond with, "that's right, come to think of it . . ." and another piece of the puzzle falls into place.

With this subjective data gathered, the doctor has a good idea of what is wrong. A differential diagnosis, a list of possibilities, is set in his mind. Now he moves into the next segment of the clinical encounter: collecting objective data.

Objective: After hearing your story and asking you specific questions, the physician now turns toward a physical exam. The purpose of the objective segment is to confirm what he already suspects. He'll know what to look for to confirm his suspicion. You're probably well aware of him feeling your pulse, listening to your breath, heart, and bowel sounds with a stethoscope, and testing the briskness of your reflexes with a reflex hammer. However, this portion of the assessment began perhaps before you made it to the exam room! Subtle cues like how you walk, the expression on your face, and how you sit are all clues he gathers and carefully considers. Consider, for example, a patient who arrives at a hospital looking sick and shuffles in slowly, not wanting to move. Their characteristic moves and expressions may tell the doctor a great deal without a word being spoken.

The physical exam is focused on the part of the body, or system, most affected. You'd expect a doctor to examine the painful toe that prompted your appointment, and he most certainly will. Then he'll expand his search, feeling and comparing other joints. He will investigate other parts of you, careful not to miss something you may not have noticed.

The physical exam often confirms what the doctor already suspects. Tests may be needed to confirm or rule out his suspicions. Suppose you go to the clinic with sudden onset of a painful, red, swollen big toe. The doctor may think gout, especially if your story is consistent with that diagnosis and you have risk factors (male, older, overweight). However, even if your symptoms fit nicely in that category, a doctor must think beyond the obvious. In this case, a close second on the doctor's differential diagnosis is an infected joint. Both would present with similar symptoms. Since an infected joint may leave permanent damage, the doctor will not want to miss it. He will likely want to take a fluid sample from the joint to look for infection or crystals.

After hearing your story and confirming his diagnosis with a physical exam and tests, he now proceeds to an assessment and plan.

Assessment: At this point, your physician puts together all the information he has at the time and makes a diagnosis; that is, he gives your condition a name. Typically, the assessment summarizes you in one or two sentences in his notes. In the case of gout, it might read as follows:

"A 52 year old overweight man with a history of hypertension controlled with a diuretic who presents with sudden onset right big toe pain, swelling and redness since waking this morning. Exam and lab workup (elevated serum uric acid level at 9.2 mg/dL and synovial fluid analysis that shows urate crystals) are consistent with acute gouty arthritis."

Plan: The final portion of the clinical encounter is the plan, or "to do" list. Depending on the complexity of your health, it can be pretty lengthy. The most pressing problems are listed first. In the case of gout, it could look like this:

1. *Acute gout attack of the right big toe*
   a. *Start naproxen*
   b. *Bed cradle*
   c. *Drink at least 2 litres fluids per day*

2. *Raised uric acid*
   a. *Start allopurinol in outpatients*

3. *Hypertension (controlled)*
   a. *Suggest GP switches furosemide to losartan*

4. *Overweight*
   a. *Refer to a dietitian for weight loss & gout dietary advice*

The plan is not limited to treating your current, most pressing problem but includes your other health problems and any adjustments that need to be made. This extensive plan helps the physician consider and remember all of your medical conditions and how they overlap and affect each part of you.

This SOAP approach is used universally among all doctors regardless of specialty or the country where they practice. When they think through a clinical problem, they approach it every time in this consistent and set order. When one doctor communicates with another about a patient, the clinical situation is presented methodically using this pattern.

Now that you are familiar with how doctors think, you will better understand the questions they are asking and information will flow more effectively in both directions.

Can I trust my doctor to make the correct diagnosis?

Although all physicians will follow the pattern we discussed, some physicians will arrive at a different assessment, and those who come up with the same assessment might have differing plans. Although there are multiple reasons why this might happen, the short answer is that no two doctors are the same, nor have they had identical clinical experiences. We must also remember that doctors are not perfect.

Most doctors practice what is referred to as "evidence-based medicine." This means that the doctors' approach to evaluating you and coming to an assessment and plan is based on the most up to date information available. Best practices are constantly evolving based on new studies. Even the most attentive and well-meaning doctors out there can't keep up with everything.

Because of the vast amount of human biology and disease that doctors are expected to know, they rely heavily on recognising patterns. No matter how straightforward it might seem, no disease behaves precisely as the textbook says it should. A saying common among doctors is, "When you hear hoofbeats, think horses, not zebras." Senior physicians will often remind their trainees that common things are, after all, common. A sore throat is usually just a sore throat, not a sign of leukaemia. This works well most of the time, but sometimes that zebra shows up.

For this reason, a physician will create a differential diagnosis in his mind while he is listening to you explain your experiences, examining you, and interpreting test results. He is looking for the horse, without forgetting there are zebras, too.

Even though a physician makes the best assessment and plan based on the information provided by you (subjective) and physical exam and tests (objective), sometimes they are vulnerable to pitfalls in the process.

First, he might fall into what is called "confirmational bias." Since doctors are used to what is familiar (the horse), they can focus only on those things that support the 'most likely' diagnosis and not give sufficient thought to the things that don't quite fit.

Second, he might fall into "diagnosis momentum." Think of a stone rolling down a mountain, gaining speed and power. Similarly, a doctor may give your problem a name (a diagnosis), and as you get passed on to another doctor, this label sticks even if it isn't a correct assessment. That first colleague's evaluation may bias their thinking. Symptoms and examination findings that aren't consistent with the diagnosis are dismissed, perspective is lost, and the correct diagnosis is not made.

Though you may feel uncomfortable guiding your doctor in the right direction to ensure you get appropriate care, remember you are an integral part of the doctor-patient relationship. Your ideas, concerns, and questions need to be heard because they make sure your doctor considers all the aspects and helps him think broadly.

Your doctors have spent years learning their trade. They refine their practice with every patient they see, every conference they go to and every journal article they read. They went into medicine because they care deeply about people and want to do the very best they can for every patient. You are likely to be in very capable hands. We wrote this book to give you the knowledge and insights you need to be an equal part of that doctor-patient relationship, make the most effective use of the brief time you have with your doctor, and get the best treatment possible.

What can you do?

Preparing for your appointment

Before your visit, jot down on a piece of paper answers to these questions:

1. Why am I seeing the doctor today?
2. How long have I had this problem? When did I first notice something was wrong?
3. How would I describe the issue (i.e. if there is pain, what kind of pain and when/where do I feel it)?
4. Has it been getting better or worse?
5. What makes it better? What makes it worse? What have I been doing for it?

In addition:

- Take a list of all your medications, including the doses, or take the medicines themselves.
- Have a list of any medical conditions you've had, past hospitalisations, and surgeries.
- When you see a new doctor for the first time, you may want to let his office know ahead of time where your medical records are so that they can send for copies. Doing this will help your physician determine how you've been treated before.

If your doctor sends you for tests

Don't hesitate to ask questions before a test. For example, you might ask:

1. What test is being done?
2. Why is it being done and what is it looking for?
3. What are the risks or dangers of the test?
4. Who will do the test?
5. What do I need to do to prepare (some tests, for example, require you not to eat beforehand?
6. What do you expect to find, and why?

Before you leave the clinic

It is vital you understand your diagnosis and the plan to address it. To get the most from your appointment:

1. You can help your physician think through your case, or reconsider a diagnosis, by asking questions about his differential diagnosis. If he feels you have condition "x", you might ask:
   - What else do you think this could be?
   - What is the worst thing among the possibilities you've considered?
2. Ask questions, even if you think it is a trivial concern. If you don't ask, the doctor will assume you understand.
   Make sure you understand:
   - What your condition is.
   - Why you have it, or what caused it.
   - What the treatment is.
   - The expected outcome.
   - Instructions you need to follow and medication or other therapy.
   - What you can do to prevent the problem from recurring.
   - What you should watch for, or if you should call the clinic when something changes.
   - When you should see the doctor again.
3. You can ask for written copy of this information. Many doctors will be happy to provide a written summary of your diagnosis and the instructions you should follow.
4. After the physician has given you instructions, re-state it back to him in your own words. You might say, "If I understand you correctly, I have .... which is caused by .... I need to ....

Chapter 49

Taking part in clinical trials of new treatments

The frontiers of medicine move forward every day. All around the world, doctors, nurses, scientists, pharmacists, statisticians, data managers and countless others strive daily to bring us better treatments.

We tend to think about the development of entirely new medicines, but that's just one aspect of this quest for better treatments. Much research goes into optimising existing drugs: finding the best dose, the modifications needed for people with other health issues, and increasing effectiveness through combinations with other medicines. Other forms of treatment are studied, too: physiotherapy, diet and nutrition, psychological therapy, social support and so on. Though studies of entirely new drugs tend to cause the most excitement, this optimisation of existing treatments can often significantly improve the benefits you get from your treatment.

Regardless of what kind of study you may be thinking of taking part in, the general principles will be the same.

Firstly, the researchers will decide precisely what the question is that they want to answer. For example:

- Is drug A better than drug B?
- What is the most effective and safe dose, A, B or C?
- Is weekly physiotherapy significantly more effective than once a month?

The researchers need to define exactly what success looks like. How much better does drug A have to be compared to drug B, 10% better, 20% better, or just no worse.

Then researchers will decide the kind of people they need to answer their research question safely. They will want to include people as similar as possible to those who would receive this treatment if proven effective. However, they also need to make sure they don't put anyone at unnecessary risk, so certain groups of people will be excluded from the study: people under or over certain ages, pregnant women, people with severe kidney or liver disease, for example. These criteria will be carefully selected based on the characteristics of the disease, and of the medicine or treatment being investigated.

The remainder of the study will then be planned. Researchers will decide on issues such as:

- For how long will the treatment be given.
- For how long will people be followed up afterwards.
- Under what circumstances will people be pulled out of the study.
- What tests will be needed to answer the question, and how often should they be done.
- How often will study participants need to be seen both to understand how well the treatment is working and ensure their safety.

Once the study has been planned, permission to conduct the study must be obtained from one or more panels of independent experts. These panels exist to ensure that studies are only allowed to take place if they will answer a valid question, not put anyone at unnecessary risk of harm, and are designed and conducted appropriately and ethically. These panels may refuse permission to conduct a study or ask for changes.

A study may be conducted in just a single hospital or clinic or at multiple sites across a country or even around the world. The staff running the trial will be trained in all aspects of the study to ensure that the same standards are applied at all sites.

Finally, the study can begin. Potential study participants can be found by searching medical records, requesting referrals from other doctors, or even advertising in newspapers or on the radio. At the first visit, researchers will explain why the study is being conducted, the risks and benefits, and what visits and tests will be required. You may be asked to sign your consent to participate in this study at that time or sent away with information to read and think about before coming back to give your written consent at the next visit.

You should understand that no benefits can be guaranteed and that there may be potential risks. However, the study team will do everything to minimise the risk. You may receive the new treatment, the old treatment, or dummy pills (placebos). In a good study, neither you nor your doctor will know what treatment you are getting until the study has finished. This is to prevent you or your doctor from having a biased assessment stemming from your expectations of the treatment.

In some countries, you may be paid to participate in certain kinds of study, but generally, all you will get is free treatment and reimbursement of your expenses. You are taking part in this study to help others and perhaps gain some benefit yourself. Generally, people taking part in studies do better than those not in studies, even if they take dummy tablets. This is most likely because of the high level of attention to their health and the frequent clinic visits.

Once the study has been completed and analysed, you will be able to find out which treatment you received, and you should be given a summary of the results. If the study was successful, you might be allowed to continue or change to the new treatment.

The phases of development for a new medicine

Discovery

Lots, perhaps tens of thousands of compounds, are screened to see if they might be useful in the disease.

Usually, this screening tests if each compound blocks a vital enzyme or binds to certain types of cell receptors.

Promising leads are then modified to make them more effective, longer-lasting, more soluble, less toxic, etc.

Eventually, the most promising compound is selected to move to the next phase.

Pre-clinical

Here the compound is tested for activity in animal models of the disease.

Its toxicity is studied in animals to see if it has unexpected or unacceptable problems.

Scientists will study how the compound is transported around the body, where it goes, and how it is removed from the body.

Chemists will look for more effective ways to produce the chemical in its purest form.

If a compound passes all of these tests, the results will be reviewed by panels of experts to see if it should move on to trials in humans.

Clinical - Phase I

Phase I is the first time the drug will be given to humans.

Usually, this will begin with healthy volunteers, but sometimes patients.

Doctors will begin giving it to one patient at a time, starting with small doses and slowly increasing.

They will measure how it is transported around the human body, where it goes, how it is excreted, and if it has any side effects.

At the end of phase I, the scientists will review all the results to see if the drug reaches the required levels in the body and if it has any side effects that make it unsuitable to continue.

Clinical - Phase II

In Phase II, the researchers work out the most appropriate dose.

Phase II is usually carried out in patients with the disease to be treated.

A small number of different doses will be tried in different groups of patients.

If the drug seems to be working, and if any side effects are acceptable, a dose will be selected for the large clinical trials that will determine if the new medicine will be approved for use in everyone.

Clinical - Phase III

These are the large studies that will show if the new medicine really works for the patients it was designed for.

The studies are also large enough to detect the common side-effects of the new medicine.

Usually there are at least two large studies, sometimes more.

Each study will have hundreds, or occasionally even thousands of participants.

The studies are typically carried out at multiple hospitals and clinics in several countries.

Registration

Once the studies have been completed, all the information from all the studies is put together and passed to the government medicines regulators in the appropriate countries. They will rigorously review all of the data, ask lots more questions, and finally decide if they will approve the new medicine for general use.

Clinical - Post registration

Even after a medicine has been approved by the regulators, further studies will be conducted.

Some countries require studies in their own country rather than accepting results from other countries.

New populations will be studied, perhaps children, the extreme elderly, people with kidney disease or pregnant women, depending on the need for the drug in these populations.

The drug may be tested to see how effective it is in different diseases.

Studies may be conducted on combinations with other drugs or in different formulations—a slow-release tablet, for example.

How can I take part in a clinical trial?

Clinical trials are much more likely to be running in a specialist clinic than from your family doctor's practice. You should ask your specialist if they know of any clinical trials you would be eligible for.

If the researchers are concerned they may not find enough suitable candidates among the patients of appropriate specialists, they may advertise their studies to the public. They will also do this if they are studying a condition for which not everyone goes to see a doctor, for example, anxiety, erectile dysfunction or dry, itchy eyes.

Information about clinical trials may also be posted to patient support group websites and forums.

The definitive list of clinical trials is run by the US National Library of Medicine and can be found at www.clinicaltrials.gov. Most significant studies worldwide will be listed here, even if they are not being conducted at sites in the US.

You can complete the simple form on the homepage as shown in Figure 39. Since you are looking for a trial to participate in, select 'Recruiting and not yet recruiting studies'.

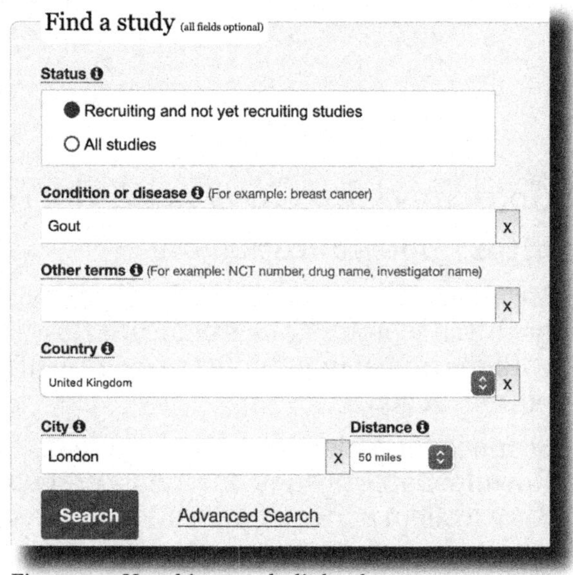

Figure 39: Use this search dialog box at www.clinicaltrials.gov to find clinical trials near you.

The search will bring up all the clinical trials that are currently looking for participants or which will start shortly. By selecting a study, you can get much more information. Such information includes which drug is being tested, how many people they need, the specific characteristics of the people they are looking for (inclusion criteria), and the characteristics of people who would not be able to participate (exclusion criteria).

The information provided can be a bit technical, but it will give you an idea of what studies are available in your region. You can then use this information to begin a conversation with your doctor.

Chapter 50

Online resources

Gout Specialists Network & The Gout Education Society

https://gouteducation.org

Mission: "The Gout Education Society is a non-profit organisation of health care professionals dedicated to raising awareness of gout arthritis, with the aim of improving the overall quality of care and minimising the burden of gout."

Sections for patients and professionals.
Downloadable posters, information sheets, trackers.
An excellent series of educational videos about many aspects of gout and its treatment.
Search facility to find a gout specialist near you (US).

The Alliance for Gout Awareness

https://www.goutalliance.org

Mission: "The Alliance for Gout Awareness works to reduce stigma and empower patients by improving public understanding of gout. Members collaborate on educational materials and support resources. By heightening public awareness and addressing common misconceptions, the Alliance for Gout Awareness emboldens patients to acknowledge the disease's impact and to seek the treatment they need.'

A useful mix of videos, podcasts, information sheets and infographics.

UK Gout Society

http://www.ukgoutsociety.org

Mission: "The UK Gout Society is a registered charity established in 2002 to provide basic information to people living with gout."

A modest website with useful gout factsheets.
Will answer questions by email.

Healthtalk

https://healthtalk.org/gout/overview

Mission: "Real People. Real-life experiences. Thousands of people have shared their experiences on film to help you understand what it's like to have a health condition such as breast cancer or arthritis."

An excellent collection of interviews on a broad range of topics with people suffering from gout.

GoutPal Gout Forum

https://goutpal.net

A broad-ranging forum where people with gout can post questions and get help, suggestions and advice from other gout sufferers.

The Gout and You Blog

https://goutandyou.com

Spiro Koulouris offers his personal take on all things gout.

The Gout Support Group Of America

https://www.facebook.com/groups/thegoutsupportgroupofaustin/

Members-only Facebook support group run by a physician and a patient advocate

New Zealand based Facebook support group

https://www.facebook.com/groups/goutarthritis

Arthritis Action

https://www.arthritisaction.org.uk

Mission: "Arthritis Action is the UK charity giving hands-on, practical help to improve the quality of life of people affected by arthritis. We offer an integrated self-management approach, which looks at both the physical and mental health impact of living with arthritis. We support people living with musculoskeletal conditions through healthy eating advice, mental health resources, pain management techniques, local groups, and exercise advice and resources. We also offer one-to-one nutritional consultations, access to clinical appointments with our network of osteopaths, physiotherapists, and acupuncturists, and a personalised pathway for goal setting through our Membership to help people take control of their arthritis and enjoy life to the full.'

Arthritis Action covers all forms of arthritis. There is not a lot of gout-specific information; however, the £20 annual membership (£15 paying by direct debit) allows access to nutritional and weight guidance from a dietitian, two subsidised appointments with an osteopath or physiotherapist, individual support, online exercise classes and a newsletter

Versus Arthritis

https://www.versusarthritis.org/

Mission: "We are Versus Arthritis. We're the 10 million people living with arthritis. We're the carers, researchers, healthcare professionals, friends, parents, runners and fundraisers, all united in our ambition to ensure that one day, no one will have to live with the pain, fatigue and isolation that arthritis causes. Alongside volunteers, healthcare professionals, researchers and friends, we do everything we can to push back against arthritis. Together, we'll continue to develop breakthrough treatments, campaign relentlessly for arthritis to be seen as a priority and support each other whenever we need it."

The organisation is not gout specific, but gout is amongst the topics covered.
Useful search facility for arthritis support groups in your area.
Online community with chatrooms and archived topics.

Arthritis Foundation

https://www.arthritis.org/home

Mission: "The Arthritis Foundation is boldly pursuing a cure for America's #1 cause of disability while championing the fight to conquer arthritis with life-changing science, resources, advocacy and community connections."

Covers many forms of arthritis but has lots of good, gout-specific information, including a few videos.
You can search for local groups and activities and clinical trials.

Creaky Joints

https://creakyjoints.org
https://creakyjoints.org.au
https://creakyjoints.ca

Mission: "Our mission at CreakyJoints is to inspire, empower and support arthritis patients to put themselves at the centre of their care by providing evidence-based education and tools that help them make informed decisions about the daily and long-term management of arthritis. We want to live our lives, despite our arthritis."

US-based site with satellites in Canada and Australia
Information, news, advocacy on all types of arthritis
Hosts The Gout Show podcast (https://creakyjoints.org/thegoutshow/)

Arthritis Australia

https://arthritisaustralia.com.au/types-of-arthritis/gout/

Mission: "Arthritis Australia is dedicated to improving quality-of-life for the millions of Australians living with arthritis through education, programs and advocacy. We also fund world-class research to increase our knowledge of arthritis and find better ways to prevent, treat and hopefully cure the condition in its many forms."

Basic information on gout.
Resources to help you find healthcare professionals and support groups near you.

Your personal data record

My healthcare team

Name:	
Position:	
☎	📱
✉	
Address:	Notes:

Name:	
Position:	
☎	📱
✉	
Address:	Notes:

Name:

Position:

Address:

Notes:

Name:

Position:

Address:

Notes:

Name:

Position:

Address:

Notes:

Name:

Position:

Address: | Notes:

Name:

Position:

Address: | Notes:

Name:

Position:

Address: | Notes:

Name:

Position:

Address:

Notes:

Name:

Position:

Address:

Notes:

Name:

Position:

Address:

Notes:

Attacks / flare-ups

Date started:	Date ended:
Joint(s) affected:	
Treatment:	
Notes:	

Date started:	Date ended:
Joint(s) affected:	
Treatment:	
Notes:	

Date started:	Date ended:
Joint(s) affected:	
Treatment:	
Notes:	

Date started:	Date ended:
Joint(s) affected:	
Treatment:	
Notes:	

Date started:	Date ended:
Joint(s) affected:	
Treatment:	
Notes:	

Date started:	Date ended:
Joint(s) affected:	
Treatment:	
Notes:	

Date started:	Date ended:
Joint(s) affected:	
Treatment:	
Notes:	

Date started:	Date ended:
Joint(s) affected:	
Treatment:	
Notes:	

Date started:	Date ended:
Joint(s) affected:	
Treatment:	
Notes:	

Date started:	Date ended:
Joint(s) affected:	
Treatment:	
Notes:	

Date started:	Date ended:
Joint(s) affected:	
Treatment:	
Notes:	

Date started:	Date ended:
Joint(s) affected:	
Treatment:	
Notes:	

Date started:	Date ended:
Joint(s) affected:	
Treatment:	
Notes:	

Date started:	Date ended:
Joint(s) affected:	
Treatment:	
Notes:	

Date started:	Date ended:
Joint(s) affected:	
Treatment:	
Notes:	

Date started:	Date ended:
Joint(s) affected:	
Treatment:	
Notes:	

Date started:	Date ended:
Joint(s) affected:	
Treatment:	
Notes:	

Date started:	Date ended:
Joint(s) affected:	
Treatment:	
Notes:	

Date started:	Date ended:
Joint(s) affected:	
Treatment:	
Notes:	

Date started:	Date ended:
Joint(s) affected:	
Treatment:	
Notes:	

Date started:	Date ended:
Joint(s) affected:	
Treatment:	
Notes:	

Date started:	Date ended:
Joint(s) affected:	
Treatment:	
Notes:	

Date started:	Date ended:
Joint(s) affected:	
Treatment:	
Notes:	

Date started: Date ended:

Joint(s) affected:

Treatment:

Notes:

Date started: Date ended:

Joint(s) affected:

Treatment:

Notes:

Date started: Date ended:

Joint(s) affected:

Treatment:

Notes:

Date started: Date ended:

Joint(s) affected:

Treatment:

Notes:

Date started: Date ended:

Joint(s) affected:

Treatment:

Notes:

Date started: Date ended:

Joint(s) affected:

Treatment:

Notes:

Medication

Name:	
Dose:	
Date started:	Date stopped:
Reason for starting:	
Reason for stopping:	
Notes:	

Name:	
Dose:	
Date started:	Date stopped:
Reason for starting:	
Reason for stopping:	
Notes:	

Name:	
Dose:	
Date started:	Date stopped:
Reason for starting:	
Reason for stopping:	
Notes:	

Name:	
Dose:	
Date started:	Date stopped:
Reason for starting:	
Reason for stopping:	
Notes:	

Name:	
Dose:	
Date started:	Date stopped:
Reason for starting:	
Reason for stopping:	
Notes:	

Name:	
Dose:	
Date started:	Date stopped:
Reason for starting:	
Reason for stopping:	
Notes:	

Name:	
Dose:	
Date started:	Date stopped:
Reason for starting:	
Reason for stopping:	
Notes:	

Name:	
Dose:	
Date started:	Date stopped:
Reason for starting:	
Reason for stopping:	
Notes:	

Name:

Dose:

Date started: Date stopped:

Reason for starting:

Reason for stopping:

Notes:

Name:

Dose:

Date started: Date stopped:

Reason for starting:

Reason for stopping:

Notes:

Name:

Dose:

Date started: Date stopped:

Reason for starting:

Reason for stopping:

Notes:

Name:	
Dose:	
Date started:	Date stopped:
Reason for starting:	
Reason for stopping:	
Notes:	

Name:	
Dose:	
Date started:	Date stopped:
Reason for starting:	
Reason for stopping:	
Notes:	

Name:	
Dose:	
Date started:	Date stopped:
Reason for starting:	
Reason for stopping:	
Notes:	

Name:

Dose:

Date started: Date stopped:

Reason for starting:

Reason for stopping:

Notes:

Name:

Dose:

Date started: Date stopped:

Reason for starting:

Reason for stopping:

Notes:

Name:

Dose:

Date started: Date stopped:

Reason for starting:

Reason for stopping:

Notes:

Uric acid blood test results

	Target uric acid level	
No tophi	≤ 6 mg/dl	(0.36 mmol/L)
Tophi present	≤ 5 mg/dl	(0.30 mmol/L)

Date	Result

Date	Result

Date	Result

Date	Result	

Tophi

Use these pages to record any tophi you may have and how they change over time. With good control of your blood uric acid levels, tophi should slowly shrink and disappear.

Location:	
Date first noticed:	
Date	Size

_ocation:	
)ate first noticed:	
)ate	Size

_ocation:	
)ate first noticed:	
)ate	Size

Location:	
Date first noticed:	
Date	Size

Location:	
Date first noticed:	
Date	Size

Location:	
Date first noticed:	
Date	Size

Location:	
Date first noticed:	
Date	Size

Doctor / clinic visits

Use these pages to plan your appointments with your doctors and other healthcare providers. Write down reminders of what you would like to talk about.

Afterwards, record what was discussed and any decisions made.

Name:	Date:
What I want to discuss	
What was discussed	
Decisions made	
Next appointment:	

Name:	Date:
What I want to discuss	
What was discussed	
Decisions made	
Next appointment:	

Name:	Date:
What I want to discuss	
What was discussed	
Decisions made	
Next appointment:	

Name:	Date:
What I want to discuss	
What was discussed	
Decisions made	
Next appointment:	

Name:	Date:
What I want to discuss	
What was discussed	
Decisions made	
Next appointment:	

Name:	Date:
What I want to discuss	
What was discussed	
Decisions made	
Next appointment:	

Name:	Date:
What I want to discuss	
What was discussed	
Decisions made	
Next appointment:	

Name:	Date:
What I want to discuss	
What was discussed	
Decisions made	
Next appointment:	

Name:	Date:
What I want to discuss	
What was discussed	
Decisions made	
Next appointment:	

Name:	Date:
What I want to discuss	
What was discussed	
Decisions made	
Next appointment:	

Name:	Date:
What I want to discuss	
What was discussed	
Decisions made	
Next appointment:	

Name:	Date:
What I want to discuss	
What was discussed	
Decisions made	
Next appointment:	

Name:	Date:
What I want to discuss	
What was discussed	
Decisions made	
Next appointment:	

Name:	Date:
What I want to discuss	
What was discussed	
Decisions made	
Next appointment:	

Name:	Date:
What I want to discuss	
What was discussed	
Decisions made	
Next appointment:	

Name:	Date:
What I want to discuss	
What was discussed	
Decisions made	
Next appointment:	

Name:	Date:
What I want to discuss	
What was discussed	
Decisions made	
Next appointment:	

Name:	Date:
What I want to discuss	
What was discussed	
Decisions made	
Next appointment:	

Name:	Date:
What I want to discuss	
What was discussed	
Decisions made	
Next appointment:	

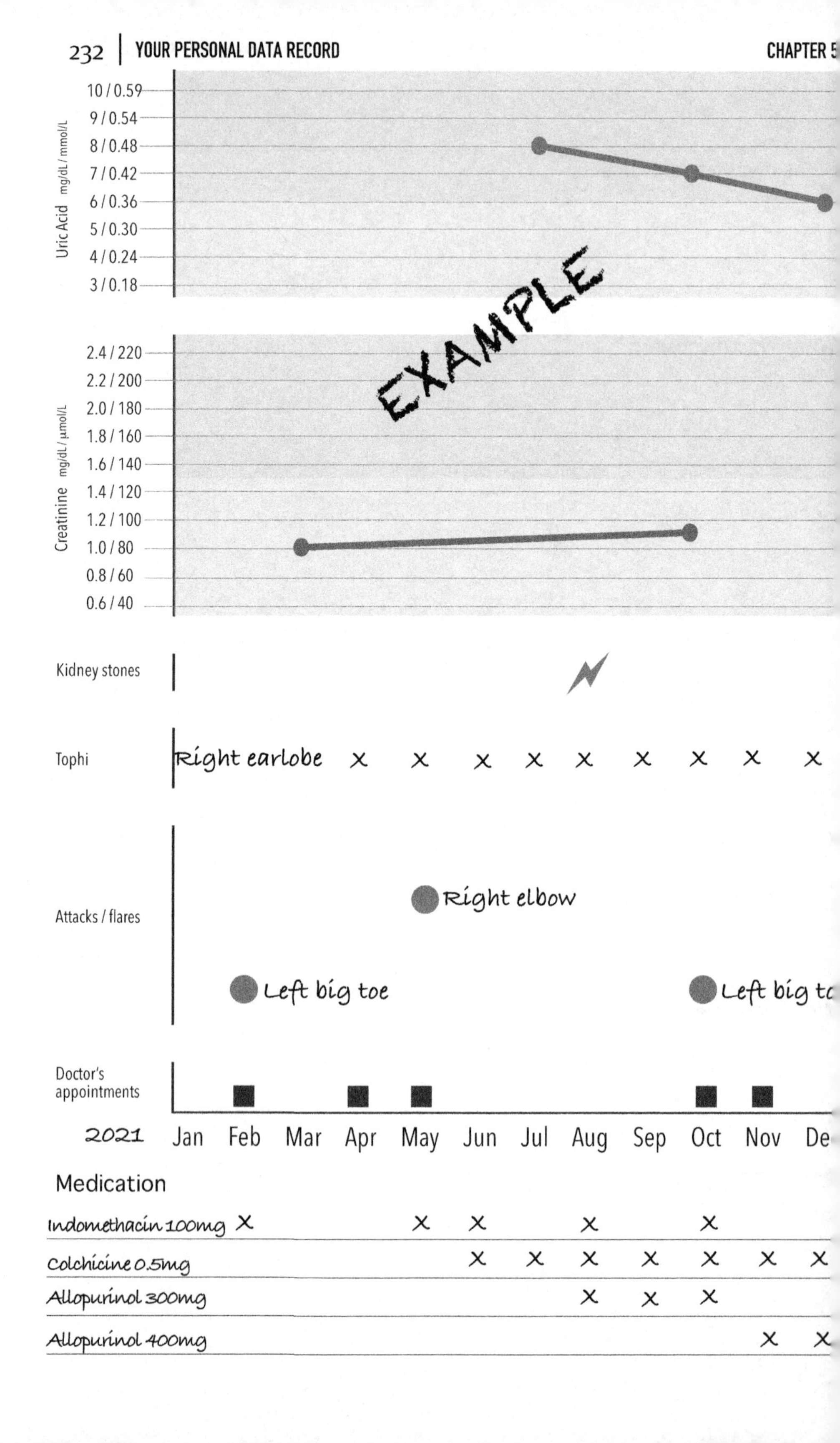
Uric Acid mg/dL / mmol/L
10 / 0.59
9 / 0.54
8 / 0.48
7 / 0.42
6 / 0.36
5 / 0.30
4 / 0.24
3 / 0.18
EXAMPLE
Creatinine mg/dL / µmol/L
2.4 / 220
2.2 / 200
2.0 / 180
1.8 / 160
1.6 / 140
1.4 / 120
1.2 / 100
1.0 / 80
0.8 / 60
0.6 / 40
Kidney stones
Tophi
Right earlobe
Attacks / flares
Right elbow
Left big toe
Left big to
Doctor's appointments
2021
Jan Feb Mar Apr May Jun Jul Aug Sep Oct Nov De
Medication
Indomethacin 100mg
Colchicine 0.5mg
Allopurinol 300mg
Allopurinol 400mg

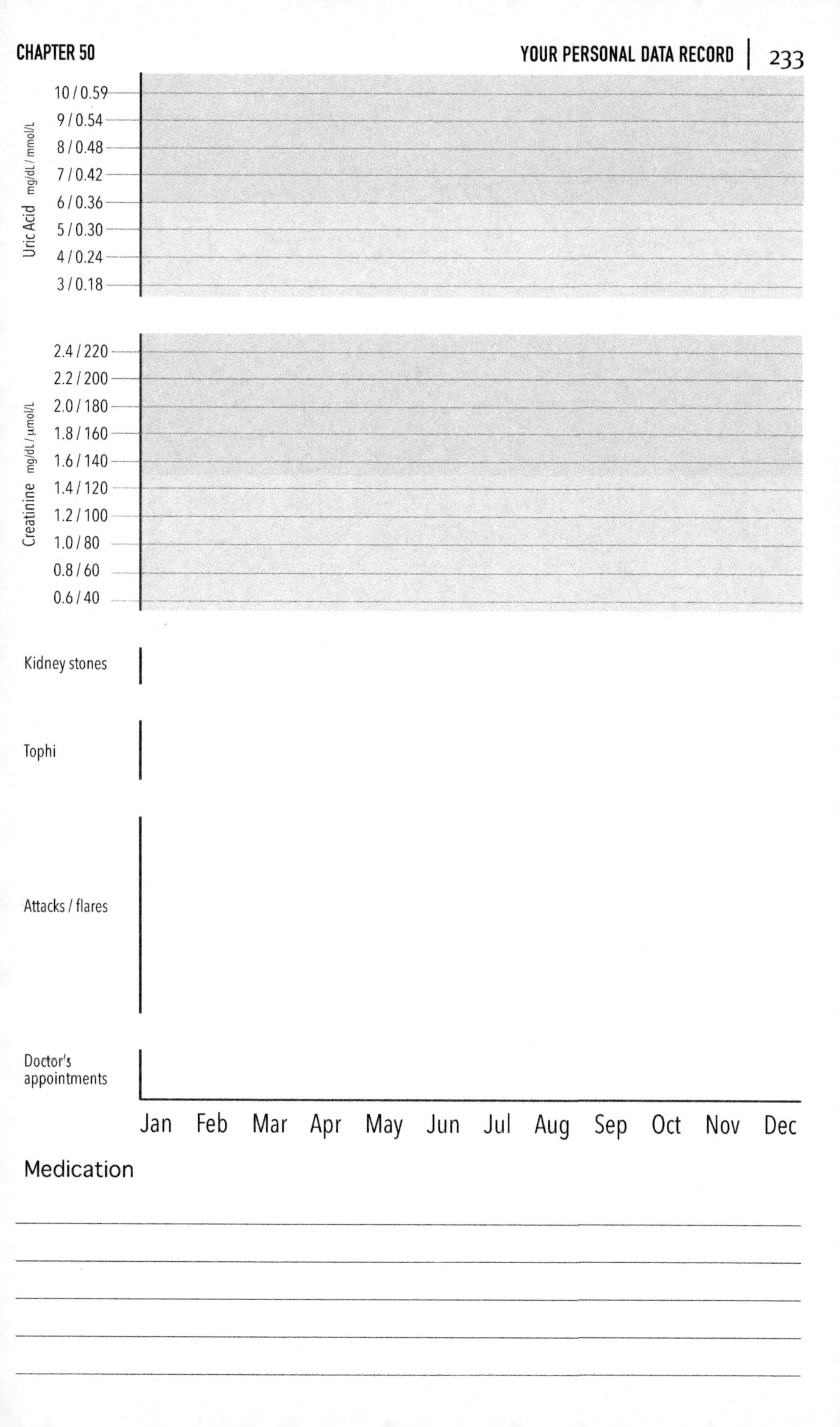
Uric Acid mg/dL / mmol/L
10 / 0.59
9 / 0.54
8 / 0.48
7 / 0.42
6 / 0.36
5 / 0.30
4 / 0.24
3 / 0.18
Creatinine mg/dL / µmol/L
2.4 / 220
2.2 / 200
2.0 / 180
1.8 / 160
1.6 / 140
1.4 / 120
1.2 / 100
1.0 / 80
0.8 / 60
0.6 / 40
Kidney stones
Tophi
Attacks / flares
Doctor's appointments
Jan
Feb
Mar
Apr
May
Jun
Jul
Aug
Sep
Oct
Nov
Dec

Medication

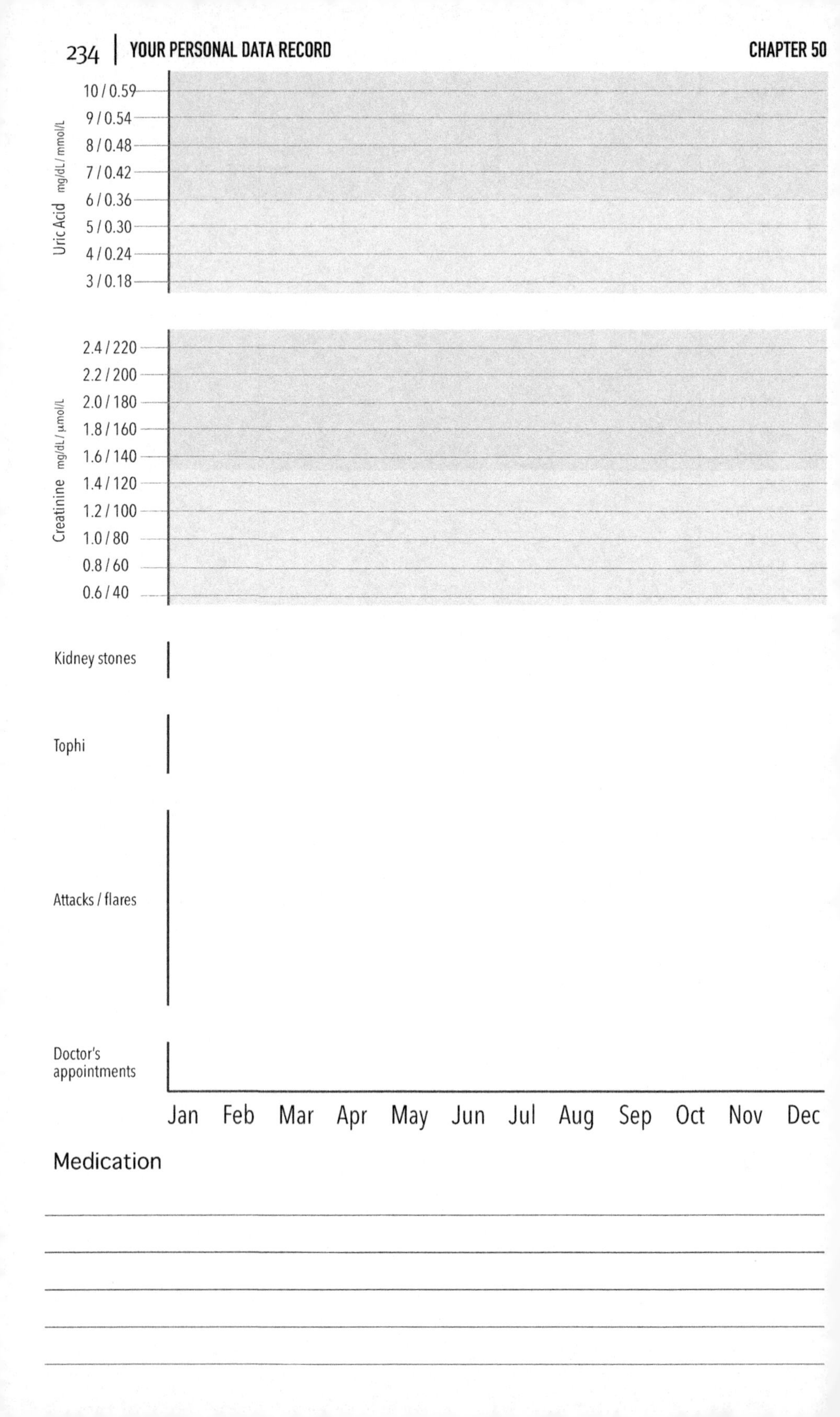
Uric Acid mg/dL / mmol/L
10 / 0.59
9 / 0.54
8 / 0.48
7 / 0.42
6 / 0.36
5 / 0.30
4 / 0.24
3 / 0.18
Creatinine mg/dL / µmol/L
2.4 / 220
2.2 / 200
2.0 / 180
1.8 / 160
1.6 / 140
1.4 / 120
1.2 / 100
1.0 / 80
0.8 / 60
0.6 / 40
Kidney stones
Tophi
Attacks / flares
Doctor's appointments
Jan
Feb
Mar
Apr
May
Jun
Jul
Aug
Sep
Oct
Nov
Dec
Medication

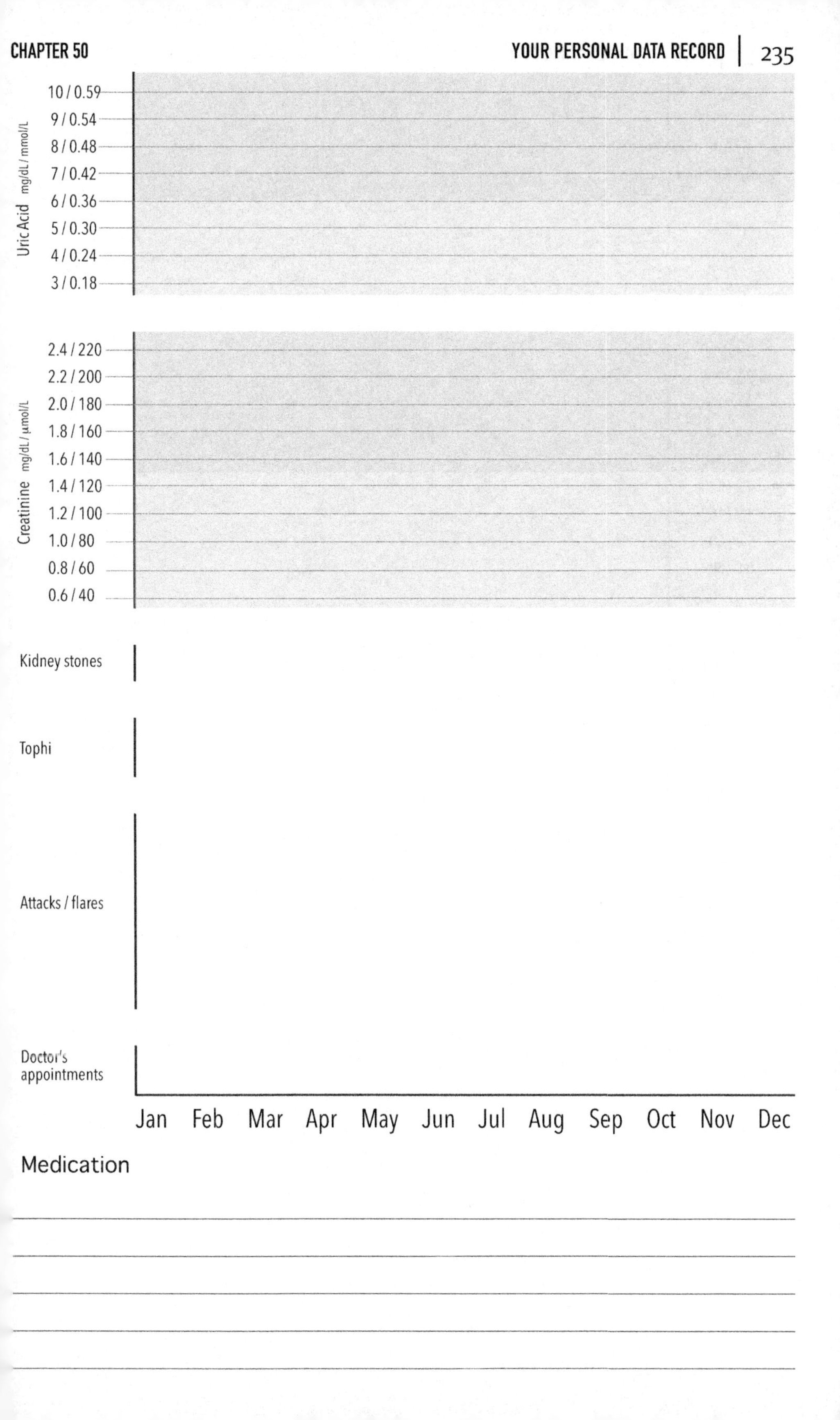
10 / 0.59
9 / 0.54
8 / 0.48
7 / 0.42
6 / 0.36
5 / 0.30
4 / 0.24
3 / 0.18
Uric Acid mg/dL / mmol/L
2.4 / 220
2.2 / 200
2.0 / 180
1.8 / 160
1.6 / 140
1.4 / 120
1.2 / 100
1.0 / 80
0.8 / 60
0.6 / 40
Creatinine mg/dL / µmol/L
Kidney stones
Tophi
Attacks / flares
Doctor's appointments
Jan Feb Mar Apr May Jun Jul Aug Sep Oct Nov Dec
Medication

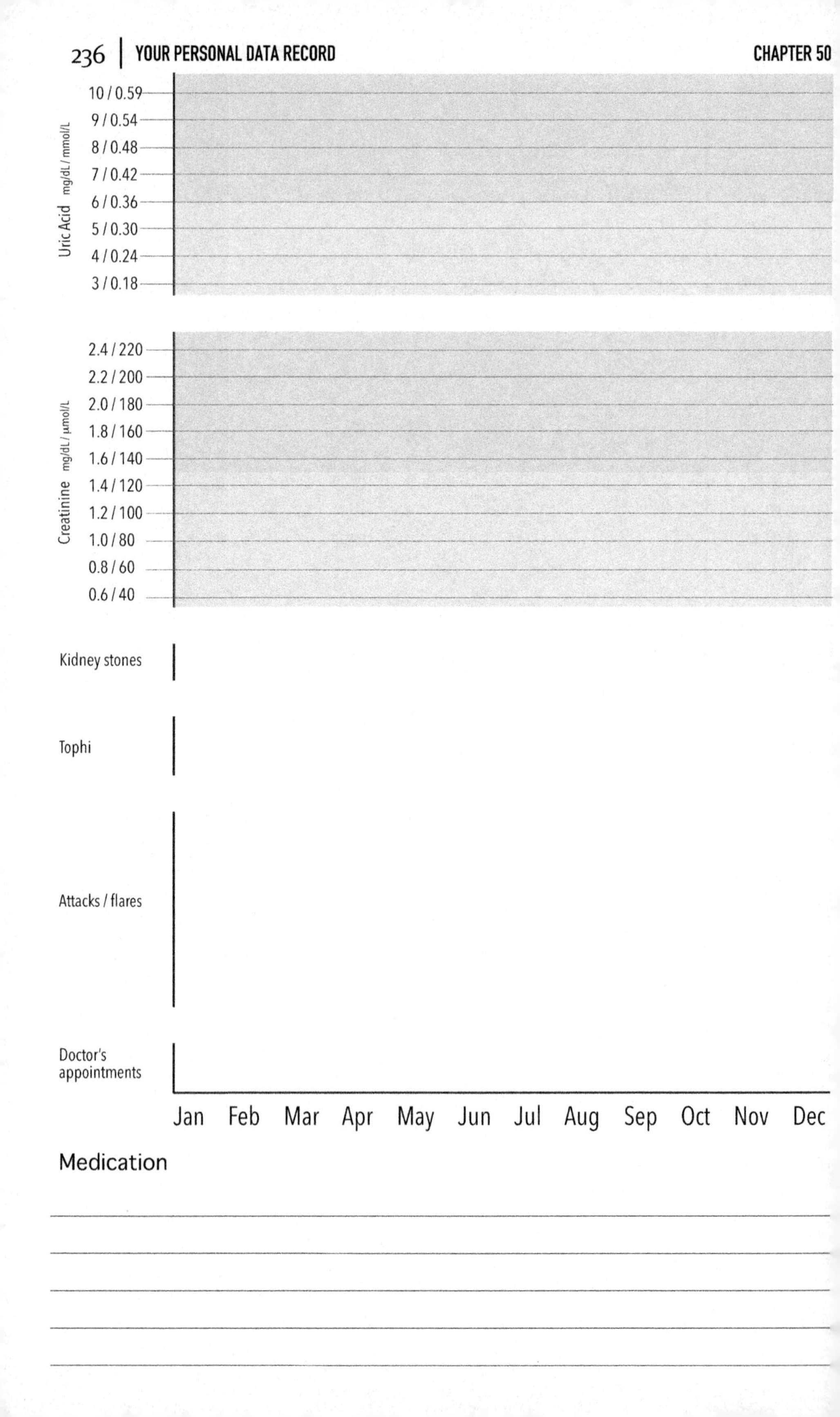
Uric Acid mg/dL / mmol/L
10 / 0.59
9 / 0.54
8 / 0.48
7 / 0.42
6 / 0.36
5 / 0.30
4 / 0.24
3 / 0.18
Creatinine mg/dL / µmol/L
2.4 / 220
2.2 / 200
2.0 / 180
1.8 / 160
1.6 / 140
1.4 / 120
1.2 / 100
1.0 / 80
0.8 / 60
0.6 / 40
Kidney stones
Tophi
Attacks / flares
Doctor's appointments
Jan
Feb
Mar
Apr
May
Jun
Jul
Aug
Sep
Oct
Nov
Dec
Medication

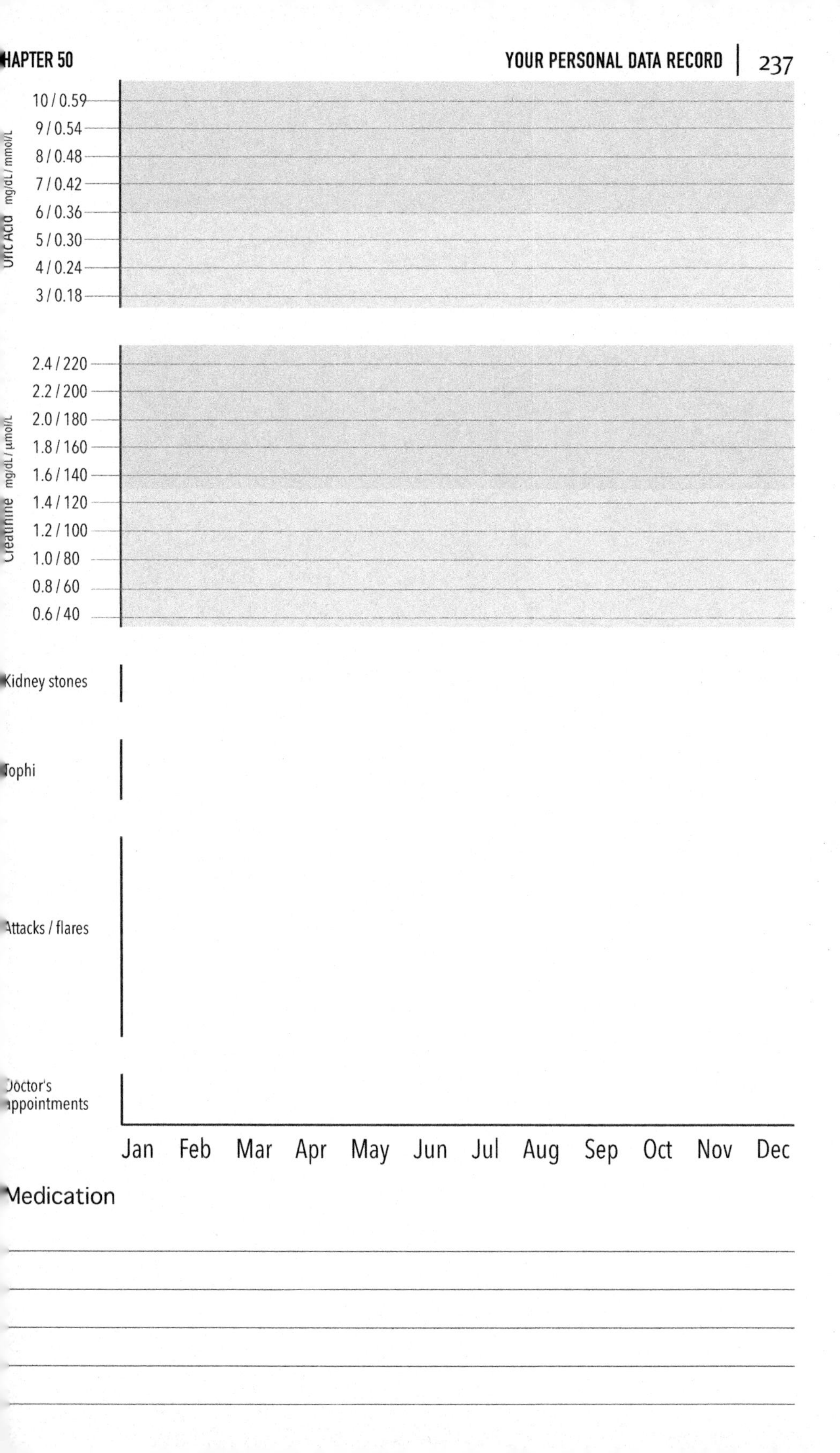
Uric Acid mg/dL / mmol/L
10 / 0.59
9 / 0.54
8 / 0.48
7 / 0.42
6 / 0.36
5 / 0.30
4 / 0.24
3 / 0.18
Creatinine mg/dL / µmol/L
2.4 / 220
2.2 / 200
2.0 / 180
1.8 / 160
1.6 / 140
1.4 / 120
1.2 / 100
1.0 / 80
0.8 / 60
0.6 / 40
Kidney stones
Tophi
Attacks / flares
Doctor's appointments
Jan Feb Mar Apr May Jun Jul Aug Sep Oct Nov Dec

Medication

Index

X

Y

Picture credits

Cover pictures:

Tophus on knee: "GoutTophiKnee" by Nick Gorton is licensed under the Creative Commons Attribution-Share Alike 3.0 Unported license. Image cropped.

Gout affecting big toe: "Gout Signs and Symptoms"by www.scientificanimations.com/ is licensed under the Creative Commons Attribution-Share Alike 4.0 International license.

Urate crystals: "Gout - monosodium urate crystals (20X, polarized, red compensator)" by Gabriel Caponetti is licensed under the Creative Commons Attribution-Share Alike 3.0 Unported license.

Erosion of finger bone: "Gicht-Arrosion am proximalen Interphalangealgelenk D4 92M - CR ap - 001 - Annotation" by Hellerhoff is licensed under the Creative Commons Attribution-Share Alike 4.0 International license.

Figure 8 on page 13: "Gout presenting in the metatarsal-phalangeal joint of the big toe" by Intermedichbo - Dr Milorad Dimić is licensed under the Creative Commons Attribution-Share Alike 4.0 International license.

Figure 9 on page 14: "Joint" by Laboratoires Servier is licensed under the Creative Commons Attribution-Share Alike 3.0 Unported license. Edited to highlight affected joints.

Figure 10 on page 14: "GoutTophiElbow" by Nick Gorton is licensed under the Creative Commons Attribution-Share Alike 3.0 Unported license.

Figure 11 on page 25: "Light microscopy of a touch preparation of a gout tophus, showing urate crystals" by Mikael Häggström is licensed under the Creative Commons Attribution-Share Alike 4.0 International license.

Figure 12 on page 25: "Calcium Oxalate Detail" by J3D3 is licensed under the Creative Commons Attribution-Share Alike 4.0 International license.

Figure 13 on page 25: "Gout - monosodium urate crystals (20X, polarized, red compensator)" by Gabriel Caponetti is licensed under the Creative Commons Attribution-Share Alike 3.0 Unported license.

Figure 16 on page 43: "GoutTophiKnee" by Nick Gorton is licensed under the Creative Commons Attribution-Share Alike 3.0 Unported license. Image cropped.

Figure 17 on page 44: "ChronicGout" by Nick Gorton is licensed under the Creative Commons Attribution-Share Alike 3.0 Unported license.

Figure 18 on page 44: "Case 30-top" by Herbert L. Fred, MD and Hendrik A. van Dijk with permission.

Man with head in hands on page 92: Adobe stock image

Glass of water on page 124: Adobe stock image.

Cherries on page 126: Adobe stock image.

Turmeric on page 126: Adobe stock image.

Frankincense on page 127: Adobe stock image.

Lemons on page 128: Adobe stock image.

Garlic on page 129: Adobe stock image.

Red chillies on page 130: Adobe stock image.

Figure 28 on page 132: "The Lacnunga" by an unknown author is in the public domain.

Figure 29 on page 133: "King Charles II." by John Michael Wright is licensed under the Creative Commons Attribution-Share Alike 4.0 International license.

igure 30 on page 134: "Pope Honorius IV" by PHGCOM is licensed under the Creative Commons ttribution-Share Alike 4.0 International license.

igure 31 on page 134: "Portrait of Benjamin Franklin" from The White House Historical Association is in ne public domain.

igure 32 on page 135: "Kublai Khan" from the National Palace Museum in Taipei is in the public domain.

igure 33 on page 135: "Portrait of a Man, Said to be Christopher Columbus" from the Metropolitan Museum of Art, NY is in the public domain.

igure 34 on page 136: "Portrait of Michel de Nostredame" by César de Nostredame is in the public omain.

igure 35 on page 137: "Samuel Johnson" by Joshua Reynolds is in the public domain.

igure 36 on page 138: "Laurel and Hardy" by Hal Roach Studios is in the public domain.

igure 37 on page 138: "Jared Leto Soho" by James Ackerley is licensed under the Creative Commons ttribution-Share Alike 3.0 Unported license.

igure 38 on page 139: "David Wells" by SD Dirk is licensed under the Creative Commons Attribution 2.0 eneric license.

octor on page 177: Adobe stock image

Finally...

rom small beginnings we hope that many more books in this Pocket Doctor eries will follow.

f you found this book helpful, please write a review for us wherever you urchased this book, or at https://thepocketdoctor.org.

hank you

en and David

can this QR code to go to The Pocket Doctor website:

Printed in Great Britain
by Amazon